15 THINGS YOUR DOCTOR DOESN'T KNOW ABOUT YOUR CHILD

Questions Answered About Developmental Delays

DR. AMBER BROOKS

Dr. Amber Brooks
14330 Midway Rd Ste 116
Dallas, TX 75244
www.dramberbrooks.com
Copyright © 2012, by Dr. Amber Brooks. All rights reserved

For more information regarding special discounts for bulk purchases, please contact office@mychildwellness.com or (469) 547-1173.

Edited by Dominique Chatterjee
Book layout and cover design by Dan Yeager
ISBN 978-0-9882758-0-5
SAN 920-4555
Library of Congress Control Number: 2012952830
Manufactured in the United States of America

Disclaimer: All the information found herein is provided for general information purposes only. The information, ideas, procedures, suggestions and material provided is not intended to diagnose or treat any condition or symptom and its use is not intended to be a substitute for medical or professional advice or diagnoses. This book contains general information about medical conditions and treatments, specific to children. The information is not advice and should not be treated as such. The medical information in this book is provided "as is" without any representations or warranties, express or implied. Dr. Amber Brooks, C.A.C.C.P. and Whole Child Wellness make no representations or warranties in relation to the medical information contained herein. Without prejudice to the generality of the foregoing paragraph, Dr. Amber Brooks does not warrant that the medical information in this book is complete, true, accurate, up-to-date, or non-misleading. Dr. Amber Brooks, C.A.C.C.P. and Whole Child Wellness specifically disclaim all warranties, either expressed or implied, statutory or otherwise, including but not limited to the implied warranties of merchantability, non-infringement and nutrition for particular purpose. Dr. Amber Brooks, C.A.C.C.P. and Whole Child Wellness is not responsible for any direct, indirect, special, punitive, incidental or consequential damage or any other damages whatsoever arising out of or in connection with the use of the information and material herein or in reliance on such information or material, including, without limitation, personal injury, wrongful death, or any other personal or pecuniary loss, whether the action is based in contract, tort, including negligence or otherwise.

Professional assistance: All matters regarding your health require medical supervision. You must not rely on the information in this book as an alternative to medical advice from your doctor or other professional healthcare provider. If you have any specific questions about any medical matter, you should consult your doctor or other professional healthcare provider. If you think you or your child may be suffering from any medical condition, you should seek immediate medical attention. You should never delay seeking medical advice, disregard medical advice, or discontinue medical treatment because of information contained in this book.

Dedication

This book is dedicated to Greg, the most amazing man I know for his undying love and support.

Acknowledgments

Since I was fifteen, I knew I wanted to be a doctor, that my calling was in pediatrics. I had been ill as a child, and doctors never seemed to listen, nor did they figure out what was wrong. Due to these experiences, I committed my life to healing children, and each day I happily come to work to fulfill my passion. I tackled writing this book to help those on a greater scale. That small town mother of four without community resources or the ability to attend conferences—this may aid her in her journey to find answers for her child. Or, for the doctor who has been chastised for asking questions, this can be a safe place to get information and open up possibilities for future healing. Thank you to everyone that was a part of my journey to fulfill another dream; no words can express my love and gratitude to you all. A special thank you to the following people:

My amazing husband and tireless cheerleader Greg for his unconditional love, his support in achieving all my goals and aspirations, picking me up on down days, and believing in me always.

My mother and biggest fan Kerrie Brooks for grooming my innate healing gifts since childhood, instilling in me that life is limitless, and encouraging me to always share my God-given gifts with the world.

My father John Groner for teaching me to fight for what I believe in, work hard, and know my destiny is in my control.

My sister Brittany Brooks and nephew Darien for always bringing joy to my life and keeping me on my toes.

Jennifer Stanton, the wind beneath my wings, trusted right-hand woman, and the person that keeps me sane every day. Without you, the parents, kids, and I would be lost. You are such a blessing.

Dr. Elena Still, my cherished friend and fellow healer, for your support, truthful feedback, and for always having a heart that understands me. You bring such joy to my life.

Betty Murray, my friend and most trusted colleague, for always answering questions, giving me the truth even when I do not want to hear it, and helping me through the maze of life. You make life simpler and always make me laugh.

Suzan Perez, my friend and healer, for nurturing my innate healing and treating me so I can be a better doctor each day for my children. You bring such peace and calm to a crazy whirlwind storm.

Angela Garcia, my friend and angel, who has been brought to me to keep perspective in place and guide me, for showing such compassion.

All of my little patients whom I adore for inspiring me to be the best. My life would be incomplete without you. I love you all so much.

All of my past, present, and future patients' parents for trusting me with your most precious gifts and for having the courage to seek guidance and wellness for your families.

All of my amazing friends, colleagues, and fellow healers for the work you do to change the lives of people every day. Thank you for your encouragement and love.

To all who read this book, each of you has helped contribute to spreading my message of healing and changing the face of medical treatment for children today and tomorrow. I am humbled and thank you with much love and gratitude.

With Love,

Dr. Brooks

Contents

Introduction:

I see many parents alone on their journey, and some days it hits me: My patients are family to me, and I am family to my patients unlike any other doctors they've known. I know about birthdays, vacations, the first visits from the tooth fairy, favorite toys, and the ins and outs of their social lives. Why? It's because I listen, understand, work from a wellness perspective—not a sickness model—and am the light that never dims but empowers them to keep going. In taking care of children, this is a large part of my day, working to give strength to a mother, explaining things so both parents and kids understand, and having "the talk" with a dad who thinks his wife is crazy for trying alternative care.

Being that constant in a family's journey can be just as challenging as it is rewarding. Patients and colleagues often ask me why I became a doctor, and my response is simple: "It chose me, pediatrics chose me, and I fulfill my purpose every day." I am a doctor and healer, and this isn't only what I do but also who I am. I have been working with children since I was fifteen in many capacities including coaching, teaching, and even working at a juvenile detention facility in college where I taught all ages of children about positive self-image, respecting themselves, and nurturing their talents to help develop positive hobbies that could occupy their time once released.

Not every child has great parents to teach and mold them, and even worse, some children are not born with the capacities to fulfill every dream that their parents had for them.

My role in life is one of service to children, children who are ignored or have lost hope. I serve my patients by being the ear that listens and the hand that heals. Mostly I enrich their lives by putting all the pieces together to solve what may be ailing them, and for children in particular, this approach can change the course of their lives. To parents, I am a source of knowledge and support, striving to treat them with respect while honoring the traditions and philosophies that ground me. Our national model of healthcare has not been designed for parents to seek alternative means of treatment, but times are changing. Yet the system cannot change fast enough as many children continue to suffer.

As you probably know by now, everyone has an opinion, and medical professionals are no different. However, experience and specialty matter when it comes to treating children. Each doctor will interpret things differently, and this is where choice comes in for parents. The key ingredient in gaining recovery or wellness is examining the child as a whole, not zeroing in on one part that is not functioning. For example, when your child has an ear infection, a general practitioner or specialist just looks at the ears. When the infections become chronic, only then do they begin to think perhaps there is a larger issue. Instead, doctors should dig down to the root of the problem when the first infection occurs and keep the child from getting recurring infections to begin with—that is the huge difference between traditional and functional medicine.

I want to share all the things parents are shocked to learn when their children are patients in my office. My mission with this book, as it is in my daily practice, is to show parents and their children how to navigate this maze of healing regardless of what stage they may be at. I am an expert in solving the problems other practitioners tell families are "not an issue," and I help families avoid wasting time and better their chances at recovery and wellness. My goal as a doctor is to see children thriving, healthy, and happy; I accomplish this in my practice by walking each family through the steps they need to take for their child individually. There is no cookie cutter way to treat children, and I do not take a cookie cutter approach in this book either. I'll highlight the things to look for and easy changes to make at home while helping you figure out what medical team to put in place for your child's healing journey. I will walk you through some of the most common things I see as contributing factors to delays and explain in detail how these issues may manifest. Toward the close of the book, I will touch upon treatment options, FAQs, and remedies you can give at home for common childhood illnesses.

You will find grey boxes labeled "Building Blocks" throughout the book. These contain clinical highlights pertaining to the information being covered and will tie the medical explanations to real-world stories and practical tips (the names have been changed for privacy). These paint a picture for parents about what other children have suffered from and describe the ways they overcame their obstacles during treatment. Before we dive in, I would like to share with you a story about one of my most memorable patients.

Building Blocks:

David was three years old when he was diagnosed with pervasive developmental delay-not otherwise specified (PDD-NOS) at two years of age. He also struggled with sleep, speech, constipation, and self-stimulatory behaviors and was compulsively eating and vomiting for no reason. The family had been to several doctors with no hope. His mom found an informational meeting to attend, and on the night she attended, I was speaking to the group. She brought David in to see me a few weeks later, and I did biomedical care (lab testing to figure out the cause of all his symptoms) and began to change his diet and add supplements. His treatment was very successful early on. Perhaps the most life-changing treatment for him was craniosacral therapy (CST).

David had craniosynostosis as an infant, so his skull bones were fused along his sutures, and the cranial bones had to be surgically cut to allow his brain room to grow. During this time, development of the brain was affected, and some of his symptoms were caused by this very early defect. Many doctors believe that children on the PDD spectrum like David suffer with smaller than normal frontal lobes, making certain developmental delays inevitable. In David's case, his frontal lobe was most affected by this procedure, and his delays may have been mostly due to this alone. CST is designed to eliminate cranial restrictions (it does not fix craniosynostosis), and with surgery like that, you can imagine he had severe restrictions throughout his craniosacral system.

After a month of CST, David began talking up a storm and slept in his own bed for the first time ever. He was dialoguing with me, asking me questions, and having long conversations. David is very bright, and I knew he was capable of healing, but the lightning speed recovery of his speech was incredible. His reading and language were above grade level for his age, and he qualified for the gifted and talented program the next school year. His compulsive eating also stopped after six weeks into care, and he made improvements socially. His bowel movements normalized, and he was not having large volume, explosive episodes anymore. I remember his mom being shocked when he began to be interested in foods he would NEVER have eaten previously, and she soon realized his picky eating days were over. David went to camp this past summer for the first time, and he had a great experience. His mom continues to see improvements all around and is just amazed at him every day. He is quite the little comedian.

If you are interested in understanding how developmental delays can be caught early and treated when found, then read on. I'll also help you figure out how to start your child on his or her journey to healing. The goal of this book is to guide you by giving manageable steps you can follow. Martin Luther King, Jr. once said, "Faith is taking the first step even when you don't see the whole staircase." If you are ready to take the next step, then I am ready to guide you. Faith, regardless of religious context, can be very powerful. So I encourage you to have faith like David's mom and open your mind to the possibilities awaiting you.

About the Author:

Dr. Amber Brooks, CACCP is a pediatric expert who has dedicated her career to changing the health of children around the world. She successfully bridges alternative and traditional medicine while providing individualized and comprehensive approaches to pediatric wellness. As a Board Certified Pediatric Chiropractor and Craniosacral Therapist, Dr. Brooks' experience is unique. She assists her patients in achieving optimal health by utilizing biomedical and functional medicine to help support their growing bodies. She has extensive experience solving complex pediatric cases and treats children worldwide. Her passion and enthusiasm for helping children has led to a fulfilling and successful career as a business owner, speaker, advocate, and mentor. Over the years, Dr. Brooks has seen the struggles across all medical modalities and has begun mentoring and consulting other physicians and practitioners who want to help children.

Through Whole Child Wellness, her private practice, she has developed specialized methods of treatment that deliver key nutritional and biomedical answers to today's pediatric health concerns: allergies, constipation, chronic ear infections, birth trauma, developmental delays, digestive problems, autism, ADD/ADHD, and nutritional and behavioral problems—all while supporting the whole child. Dr. Brooks truly understands the triumphs and tribulations of working in the realms of both traditional and alternative medicine. She has a unique perspective; her focus is on diagnosing the cause of the problem rather than treating the symptoms. Dr. Brooks has seen remarkable results on a variety of disorders and looks forward to helping you on your road to wellness!

15 Things
Your Doctor Doesn't Know About Your Child

1. Certain genetic factors increase a child's likelihood of developing a delay. (Chapter 1)

2. There are an abundant amount of benefits to functional and biomedical interventions. Families should explore how these interventions can heal their children.

3. Medicating with antibiotics in infancy can significantly impact gut integrity, and thus the immune system, leading to developmental delays. (Chapter 2: Immune System)

4. Craniosacral therapy (CST) is a useful therapy for mothers who experience breastfeeding difficulties. (Chapter 2: Role of Breast Milk)

5. Introducing rice cereal to your infant is a poor choice as it is irritating to the digestive system. (Chapter 2: Rice Cereal)

6. The foods that a child may be "sensitive" to contribute to poor behavior, delays, and inflammation. Avoiding irritating foods can avoid possible developmental delays. (Chapter 4)

7. Developmental delays don't need to be diagnosed to seek treatment. Early intervention is key! (Chapter 5)

8. The health of the gut is a critical factor of developmental delays in children. (Chapter 6)

9. Yeast is rampant among children and is underdiagnosed and undertreated, contributing to developmental delays and ongoing symptoms, including delayed speech, various behavioral problems, and eczema. (Chapter 6: The Yeast Connection)

10. The Four Red Flags are important for parents and doctors to watch for to detect early signs of trouble. (Chapter 7)

11. Daily bowel movements are important. Without them, a child may have poor behavior, picky eating, and trouble potty training. (Chapter 7)

12. Proper lab testing can change a child's life and in turn their development. Not finding the underlying cause of delays and common symptoms leaves children suffering. (Chapter 9)

13. Recovery IS possible. (Chapter 10)

14. Alternative treatment options exist and are effective in healing children. (Chapter 11)

15. Common poisons seen in vaccines, foods, and daily cleaners DO affect development. (Chapter 13)

Chapter 1: The Beginning, Genetics

It would be nearly impossible to find a person who does not know a child with a developmental delay, and yet our society continues to shove these kids in a corner with no hope for recovery. On the opposite side are parents struggling to keep their healthy children free of medications or vaccinations to avoid the chances of a delay and are left being kicked out of their pediatrician's office for challenging the establishment. This is wrong, and parents are looking for answers. The consensus varies when you poll people about the cause of developmental delays, and many traditional doctors like to solely blame genetics. This keeps children from attaining any sort of recovery, but recovery is possible.

For example, if you go to your pediatrician complaining of attention issues in your child and also report that the father has been diagnosed with attention deficit hyperactivity disorder (ADHD), the most likely conclusion will be that your child gets the ADHD diagnosis too and is prescribed medication without proper evaluation. This is how and why so many children are medicated unnecessarily and in turn respond wonderfully to alternative treatments such as biomedical care. It would be easy to chalk all developmental delays up to genetics; then doctors could just medicate. But genetics alone are simply not the answer, and ignoring the real cause only breeds a bigger issue.

Society has seen this bigger issue when examining the history of autism. Prior to 1980, finding autism was rare at 2 to 5 cases per 10,000 people. The rate is now 1 per 88 children and 1 in every 54 boys, and the medical community is frantically running around trying to figure out what went wrong. Autism is no different than any other delay in that early signs are always present, often ignored, and could have been repaired prior to diagnosis. If doctors and parents can recognize early symptoms that trigger developmental delays, they can then prevent and rid the body of the problem. Most parents know about common delays such as autism, ADD, and ADHD, but what about things like recurring ear infections, chronic constipation, or acid reflux? The latter three are considered a normal part of childhood, but are they really? No, these are not normal issues for anyone, and I will discuss throughout the book how these early signs can shed light on the entire body's functioning, thus leading to developmental delays as children grow.

Having a child is a journey from the very beginning. Regardless of all that happens, every parent has their own story and each child their own journey. I have found that most parents do best when they have easy steps to follow. These steps begin at conception and continue on throughout your child's life. As a mother, some of the most important times in life are during pregnancy, and this is a pivotal time to put your best foot forward. Many mothers will eat better, as well as cut out caffeine and alcohol for the health and safety of their precious gift. The old saying "the apple doesn't fall far from the tree" really is most appropriate here. The genetic makeup that parents pass down to their children can be a big player when it comes to growth and development. You can also learn from previous children you have had, and in some cases, delays can be avoided altogether. It is important to remember that genetics is not the whole picture; it is one of many factors that will be discussed throughout the book.

When people talk about the link between genetics and developmental delays, they are specifically referring to the numerous studies done on this particular subject. For example, several studies have reported that women who have an autoimmune disorder, or have it in their direct lineage (mother, father, sibling), have an increased chance of having a developmentally delayed child, specifically one with autism. Related conditions include lupus, adult onset rheumatoid arthritis, type 1 diabetes, hypothyroid, Hashimoto's thyroiditis, and rheumatic fever.

The abnormal amount of inflammation one's body endures with an autoimmune disorder does not allow the body to function properly. These dysfunctions often present with abnormal digestion and detoxification as well. When these autoimmune conditions exist, the body is not functioning at its peak potential. The symptoms can range widely, and the dysfunctions follow, which most importantly may affect both mother and child. For example, detoxification problems in a mom lead to the inability for her fetus to function optimally. Food, vaccines, illness, and digestion all have their part in detoxification. Adults, including pregnant women, are great at rationalizing why they may not feel good and often ignore the warning signs. The exact problem may not come to complete awareness until the child has been born and is struggling.

My advice to any family is to find a functional medicine or biomedical doctor to guide you and your family throughout every phase of life, ensuring the best chances of a healthy journey. You do not need to be suffering, ill, or delayed to have these types of doctors as your primary doctors; they are always looking to keep wellness at the forefront by proactively avoiding illness.

Building Blocks:

Functional medicine: According to the Institute for Functional Medicine, "Functional medicine addresses the underlying causes of disease, using a systems-oriented approach and engaging both patient and practitioner in a therapeutic partnership. Functional medicine addresses the whole person, not just an isolated set of symptoms. Functional medicine practitioners spend time with their patients, listening to their histories, and looking at the interactions among genetic, environmental, and lifestyle factors that can influence long-term health and complex, chronic disease."

Biomedical: The biomedical approach is based on the latest scientific research showing biological causes for developmental delays and other ailments. These causes include heavy metal poisoning, yeast infection, food sensitivity, and nutritional deficiency. This approach focuses on the root causes of an ailment, addressing the whole person rather than compartmentalizing problems. Biomedical doctors spend more time with their patients than traditional doctors, taking care to listen and look for connections between genetic, environmental, and lifestyle factors that can affect health and contribute to chronic disease.

Traditional or Allopathic medicine: This is a traditional disease-centered medical practice, where very little time is spent with patients and the underlying causes are rarely addressed. The focus is symptom or complaint relief, offering short-term care versus long-term care.

Ongoing research is happening all the time to further the fields of functional and biological medicine, and it is important to remember that genetics is only one piece of the puzzle. Many of the developmental delays examined in the following chapters can be helped; this means if you know what to look for, then you will know who to seek out for help with healing your child. If you are early in reading this book and are pregnant or thinking about becoming pregnant, this is a key opportunity for you to get started—before your child has already developed conditions that lead to delays—and to interview potential doctors to help you on your exciting new journey.

Chapter 2: Early Interventions in Infancy

Each of us does our best when approaching situations in life, especially when it comes to our children. When a child has a problem or issue and a tough decision has to be made, parents are often not sure what to do. Just as parents teach their kids to put one foot in front of the other when they begin to walk, they need to apply that philosophy to their own lives and take action. Some parents get inundated with information on what their child may be suffering from and have no idea which way to go. Without action, simple things turn into difficult things, and nothing gets accomplished. Because their children are suffering, many parents are spending sleepless nights searching for answers to what ails them. Unfortunately, parents have good reason to be alarmed: Statistics show that 1 in every 6 children have a developmental delay.

Most all parents know when something is wrong, even when they are told time and time again that their child will outgrow it. The reality is that these issues are not a phase but are in most cases true medical problems, so that parental gut instinct is right on target. Part of the problem is that, although parents try their best to find answers, they end up spending their time researching in the wrong places or bouncing from doctor to doctor instead of identifying and treating the core problem.

It is easy for parents and caregivers to get paralyzed by a diagnosis or the lack of support in their community. Of course many parents are troubled by all the whys and whats; then days turn into years, and no progress has been made. But no matter what, the answer to a child suffering is early intervention. It can save a child from ever getting labeled with a diagnosis, can keep them from chronic illness, and can increase their chances at living a long, healthy life. In explaining early interventions, it is important to get through some dense medical jargon so you have a real understanding of where this all begins. Bear with me because this is the foundation a body is built on, and a strong foundation must exist for anything to survive. That includes buildings and companies, and it holds true for the body too.

The Immune System

Let's go all the way back to the neonatal period (birth to 28 days). This is a critical time with regard to priming the gut for allergic disease. After birth, the intestinal barriers and immune system are poorly developed because they are brand new. This is important because 70% of the immune system is in the gut, and the immune and digestive systems need one another to develop, flourish, and succeed. The neonatal period is a time for normal beneficial microbial flora to develop, most commonly via breastfeeding.

Mucus membranes line all the body cavities, and they are bombarded immediately after birth by a large variety of microorganisms and proteins from the environment. The mucosal surface is huge—200 times the surface of the skin—and provides a line of defense against invaders. This is your body's personal army. Two armies of the mucosal immune system need to develop: IgA and IgM, which work together to balance the system. IgA and IgM are both antibodies that keep balance in the system by specifically working to modulate or inhibit the colonization of microorganisms and decrease the ability of dangerous agents to get into the mucosal layers. IgM is called the oral tolerance; this is induced via the gut against food antigens (a substance that evokes the production of one or more antibodies). When IgM is triggered again and again, it is likely to cause food allergies and sensitivities.

IgA is the more abundant of these two antibodies present in the mucosal linings, and it is also a crucial antimicrobial component found in breast milk. It is the first line of defense in the gastrointestinal (GI) mucosa. When something goes wrong, IgA is released to help. For example, when the GI tract gets inflamed and upset, the IgA army departs to the problem site to see what is happening and attempts to repair the area. The problem with the army going out too often is that the troops diminish in battle, and the reduction of the IgA army leads to greater chances of leaky gut, food allergies, and eczema developing.

The optimal mucosal barrier in an infant depends on adequate supply of breast milk, particularly in relation to infections, and it also plays a significant role in protecting against allergic reactions to food. It takes up to three months after birth for IgA to increase to adult values. It has been reported that those infants born to parents with low IgA show an increased prevalence of developing allergies, ear infections, and eczema. For example, studies have found cow milk allergies to be more prevalent among children whose mothers had a low level of IgA antibodies to bovine proteins. This means that the natural antibodies to cow's milk obtained from breastfeeding were not passed down as readily because the mother herself had low IgA, causing the child's body to respond with an allergy to cow milk. There is an ever-increasing number of children diagnosed with milk sensitivities, and IgA may explain how it all began. If your child is past weaning and you are struggling, there is much that can be done to mediate this immune response. The details are vast, but know that the imbalance within the system can be resolved. Parents must make dietary changes and add supplements to help the immune system recover, but this is a small thing to do to have their children's bodies functioning optimally again.

Achieving optimal flora in the gut and balance of IgA and IgM in the body is difficult for children today. As they grow and develop, they are given several rounds of antibiotics to treat various infections, and the antibiotics significantly impact the establishment of microflora as well as gut integrity. The resulting imbalance in the developing immune system can have long-term detrimental effects if not supported properly. How can this be counteracted? If your child is suffering with depleted intestinal microflora, meaning not enough "good bacteria," the introduction of probiotics will help build the bacteria levels, thereby improving the gut and immune system. It has been shown that children with atopic eczema can have a 50% reduction of symptoms by the age of two years when receiving the probiotic strain *lactobacillus*.

Unfortunately, achieving proper balance of IgA and IgM is not as simple as giving a probiotic. The role of nutrition is vital for growth and development in children. Many adults have seen improvements in their autoimmune and inflammatory conditions through making simple changes to their diets. Food can be healing, and it can be harmful; foods that appear healthy can still be harmful to someone with a food sensitivity or allergy to them.

A child's development has important correlations to food, specifically inflammatory foods, or foods that irritate the digestive system. Food can cause inflammation in the gut, and over time the inflammation works its way up through the digestive system to the neurological system. The impact on the neurological system can be vast, and many times the signs and symptoms of a developmental delay are seen as a result of this inflammation. The symptoms can include and are not limited to speech delays, tics, seizures, attention issues, impulsiveness, and learning disabilities.

Children's introduction to nutrition is most commonly taught using the food pyramid, which is outdated. The food pyramid does not take into account the newer science behind irritating foods and how they affect the digestive system. This may not seem like a big deal, but for children, the introduction to foods, particularly what they're raised on, can damage them if using this model. Old habits die hard, and the food pyramid learned in grade school will continue to be available to most people. Luckily most parents are informed and are paying closer attention to nutrition than previous generations, but there is always room for improvement. The role of food will be covered in-depth in Chapters 2 and 3, and nutrition is discussed as part of a treatment plan in Chapter 11.

The Role of Breast Milk

I often find that early interventions such as breastfeeding and proper introduction of first foods are the best insurance for a healthy child. The rates of breastfeeding are actually increasing nationwide, which gives greater hope to future generations. Although mothers are told "breast is best," they are not educated on why this is so important, nor do they know what to do when they struggle. The only option many of them have is to quit nursing, and then many children lose out on its many benefits. Our bodies are designed to function on breast milk alone until six months of age. From breast milk, an infant gets all the nutrition, fat, immune protection, and vitamins needed to ensure proper growth while their digestive systems prepare for solids.

When I meet a mother who is struggling with breastfeeding or see a breastfed infant who seems to be uncomfortable, I usually ask Mom what she is eating. By looking at her diet, I can analyze foods that could be affecting her infant's comfort and can also see what she may be feeding her infant. I also examine the infant to determine if there are any cranial restrictions that can be helped with craniosacral therapy (CST) to relieve them of pain. I have yet to treat a newborn who did not have some level of cranial restriction due to the birth or in utero constraint, and this can be painful for any child once they become symptomatic. Therefore, my advice is to bring your infant for a CST evaluation as soon as you are ready to leave the house. Most infants will become symptomatic between 4–6 weeks regardless of your birth experience (cesarean or natural birth). Taking care of these restrictions early may save your child from experiencing colic, sleepless nights, and other discomfort.

Building Blocks

A young new mother came to me with her baby girl, Cora. Cora was about five weeks old and was not breastfeeding enough, and her mom was scared. She had consulted with her OB/GYN and her lactation consultant, who helped her with positioning, but the latch was just "lazy" according to Mom. She was at the point where she was not producing as much milk and was looking for a formula option. I performed craniosacral therapy (CST) and a chiropractic adjustment on Cora, which together relieved her body tension and allowed additional comfort. Upon examining Cora, I found her suck to be very weak due to her vomer, a bone at the roof of her mouth, being stuck. When a bone in the cranium is stuck, it does not move as it should, and I can feel that restriction with my fingers upon examination. Most of these bones get stuck in the birthing process. The restrictions can make it extremely uncomfortable for a child to latch appropriately and can feel similar to a sinus headache. The more a child sucks, the more it hurts, so breastfeeding becomes very hard to do, whereas the bottle just flows formula into the mouth. I saw Cora twice a week for two weeks, and by the second visit she was latching better because the restrictions were being eliminated with CST. With early intervention, this mom was able to continue breastfeeding, which makes for a healthier and happier baby all around.

Many women will give up breastfeeding when their child has difficulties, but I have found that the following foods have a higher sensitivity in infants and may yield digestive discomfort, gas, sleeping trouble, colic symptoms, and constipation or diarrhea.

- Beans
- Broccoli
- Cabbage
- Caffeine
- Chocolate
- Citrus fruits
- Cow's milk
- Cucumbers
- Eggs
- Fish
- Garlic
- Nuts
- Onions
- Wheat

This list is not all-inclusive as every mother and child is different. Take a look at the list to see if you are consuming any of these items regularly, and start with eliminating those for a few days to see if there is an improvement. This also may be a good time for moms to be checked for food allergies. I have seen many mothers who were unaware of their food allergies and sensitivities until they began nursing and the effects were seen in their infants. Also make sure to drink plenty of water as you are taking in water for two.

If you are looking for options because you cannot breastfeed or have chosen not to breastfeed, here's a quick breakdown of formula alternatives:

1. **Goat Milk:** This is a great substitute and my favorite option (after breastfeeding, of course). It is easy to obtain, as close to human breast milk as possible, and will digest wonderfully. What makes goat milk easier to digest is that it does not contain the substance agglutinin, which causes particles to coagulate to form a thickened mass, and as a result the fat globules do not cluster together, making them easier to digest. The most common concern parents have is about the casein content. The milk proteins called casein are present in both cow and goat milks, but they actually differ. Cow milk primarily has something called alpha-s1, and this has been identified as the major allergen in cow milk. Goat milk's major casein sources are called alpha-s2 and beta-caseins. These are not among the major allergens and are usually tolerated well. Goat milk has less lactose and higher mineral content, but does lack in some areas including folic acid. Make sure to buy goat milk certified "free of bovine growth hormone (BGH) and antibiotics." Consult with your doctor before switching to goat milk. Most physicians have their own goat milk recipes that contain added ingredients to ensure that the infant receives all the necessary nutrients.

2. **Hypoallergenic Formula:** I recommend this only to those children under the age of one who seem to have a casein reaction. Casein, a milk protein, is irritating to a large number of children, and therefore some parents have to switch to formula. Not all formulas are the same, and the majorities are soy and dairy-based. Make sure you read the label. Even when it says "hypoallergenic," you want to find one that is free of casein, gluten, and soy. Most formulas also contain whey protein; this is a casein source and should be avoided by those with potential casein sensitivity. I suggest parents look into a product like Neocate, which meets all the criteria and may be covered under insurance if prescribed by a physician.

3. **Coconut Milk:** This option is best to introduce after one year. It has medium-chain triglycerides (MCT), which come from coconut oil and are a good source of essential fatty acids that the body needs. MCTs have been added to formulas for decades because they have nutritional and digestive healing benefits. This is also a fantastic option for pregnant mothers to incorporate into their diet for its natural antimicrobial and healing potential and because it contains good fat needed for fetal growth. For added benefits, also cook with coconut oil and purchase products made from coconut, such as ice cream and yogurt (kefir).

4. **Rice Milk:** Wait until after two years of age to use this substitute, and consult with your doctor before adding it to your child's diet. Make sure it is fortified, organic, and not low- or non-fat since fat is needed for the developing brain. Selecting an organic brand is important because inorganic rice milk contains much higher levels of arsenic, which can have negative effects on your child's development. This option is low in protein, so make sure you are including other sources of protein in meals.

5. **Almond Milk:** This is not a good substitute for infants because it lacks the nutritional value needed for proper growth. If you choose to add this to your child's diet later in life, please be cautious if you have an allergy to tree nuts or if one is suspected in your child. I have also noticed hyperactivity as a side effect, so eliminate this option if your child is struggling with hyperactivity.

6. **Soy Milk or Soy-based Formula:** This is my least favorite option. There are many problems with soy as your primary substitute, the first being that it is difficult to digest. Most mothers who have tried it report that their child had issues with bowel movements and discomfort. It also irritates the gastrointestinal tract, blocks

absorption of vitamins and minerals, interrupts endocrine function (by adding estrogen), and decreases thyroid function. In today's world of options, do yourself a favor and pass on soy.

7. **Dairy-based Formula:** Most parents try this route first. As discussed earlier, the milk protein called casein, specifically alpha-s1, is found in high levels in cow milk and has been identified as the major allergen in cow milk. This tends to irritate the digestive system because it is difficult to digest and can lead to many other issues, as discussed above.

8. **Raw Milk:** This has recently become a popular option for children past weaning, and I have found that just as many children tolerate it as don't. The main reason children have a bad reaction is because there is casein in raw milk too. My suggestion here is to proceed with caution due to the milk protein content and perhaps look to other options until you are sure your child can digest it.

Pediatric nutrition via breastfeeding and the proper introduction of first foods is very important; not doing either of these can often explain why children have digestive issues. Regardless of the age of your child, this is an important concept to understand because it could help explain why your child is having trouble at a later age.

The Trouble with Rice Cereal

Most of us were introduced to solids with rice cereal, and to this day new mothers are told to start with this digestively irritating food. This trend became popular in the 1930s during the Great Depression and WWII. Many were struggling financially, and for the first time women were going to work outside the home. This created a need for something inexpensive and filling, so the use of rice cereal began. It was inexpensive and kept babies full while their mothers were away working, making it a staple in every baby's diet. Our mothers and grandmothers have continued to use it almost out of habit. Unfortunately, this habit has been potentially harmful and should be broken.

The problems with rice cereal are that it is processed, difficult to digest, and lacks the nutritional value needed for growth. Many people like the iron that rice cereal offers because as the body matures it loses its iron stores, but rice cereal lacks the components needed to digest and utilize the iron, which is why constipation is usually the first complaint when rice cereal is introduced. This is important to know because undigested iron that is not used by the body can feed pathogenic (bad) bacteria that reside in the gut. If the bad bacteria grow, this will affect the immune system. Remember, 70% of the immune system resides in the gut. The activation of the immune system leads to illness, chronic infections, leaky gut, digestive inflammation, and increased risk of yeast infections. Your child will get the iron needed from mom's milk or formula, so there is no need for rice cereal. In addition, infants are not equipped with the enzymes to break down the carbohydrates in the rice cereal, making it hard to digest, and as a result many mothers report constipation, gas, and discomfort in their infants.

Through the years I have told parents to keep rice cereal out of their child's diet altogether. In most cases, children are ready for carbohydrates when they have their first teeth, a sign that the body is ready with the necessary enzymes to break down more complex foods. I prefer that a child remain off grains until age two, as most do not have proper pancreatic and digestive enzymes to adequately break down grain.

Building Blocks:

Baby Jackson was eleven months when he and his mother came to me in search of relief for his long-standing eczema. Eczema is a chronic skin condition that has an array of appearances, and the creams and ointments usually prescribed do not heal it, only treating the symptoms. Jackson had eczema since he was born, and no creams, medications, or bath remedies seemed to give him relief. Upon taking his history, I learned that his mom began him on solids at four months because he would not sleep through the night and her pediatrician told her it was because he was hungry. In an effort to keep him satisfied, she began feeding him rice cereal in addition to his soy formula. She was unable to breastfeed because he refused to latch and moved him to a soy formula recommended to her at four weeks of age. His eczema was on his chest, legs, and arms, but came and went with no explanation. In addition to his eczema, he was constipated, and his mom reported that he had colic for the first three months. I was able to remove the rice cereal and soy formula. The parents and I decided on a hypoallergenic formula, and I walked her through how to introduce first foods properly, leaving out the irritating grains. These simple changes reduced the irritation in his digestive tract that was causing trouble with bowel movements and eczema. When the inflammatory foods that cause eczema are reduced, improvements can be seen in many cases. Jackson's mother reported improved bowel movements, comfort, and the clearing of his eczema—all from simple dietary changes. Not all children need drastic measures or testing, but starting with simple changes will help you determine the next best step.

Signs of Digestive Discomfort

The term constipation is subjective, and many pediatricians will tell parents not to worry if their child has a bowel movement only three times a week or less. However, there is reason for concern. An infant, especially a breastfed infant, should have several bowel movements daily. If not, a new food or recent formula change could be a problem, and in some cases, this is the beginning of digestive issues. Either way, it is recommended to see a doctor for this to get help determining the best course of action. If you are breastfeeding, eliminate dairy for a week or two and see if your infant's bowels improve. Dairy tends to be binding for many infants. If you are formula feeding, look to eliminate dairy- or soy-based formula as both are known to be irritating to children. Look for hypoallergenic formulas such as Neocate that are free of all common irritants. Always make sure to check the labels of these so called "hypoallergenic" formulas as many contain casein (dairy protein) and may still irritate your child.

Most children will experience abnormal bowel movements or infrequent bowel movements when they have digestive issues. There are a few other signs that an infant is having digestive discomfort. First look for "fisting," when they clench their fists really tight and don't seem to relax them. Some will also hold their arms very close to their chest, making it hard to change their clothing. Another sign is when they pull their knees to their chest in a ball position; a parent may struggle to get them to stretch out, or the infant may fuss when you try. Fisting and pulling up of the knees are both signs of overall discomfort seen in infants, usually beginning in the first few weeks of life or when they have had changes to their diet. If you see either of these signs, please consult a pediatric chiropractor (www. ICPA4kids.com) to help with craniosacral restrictions and an adjustment. I have found craniosacral therapy (CST) to be invaluable for these little ones.

Building Blocks:

Some years ago I had the privilege of caring for a very small addition to the world. Casey was born six weeks premature and was having trouble nursing from the start. When a baby is in the NICU for a long period of time, they are often hooked up to several food sources, medicines, and breathing machines. Although this saves many lives, the equipment limits cranial movement, maturation of the suck-swallow reflex, and bonding. I was able to treat Casey as soon as he was released from the hospital and immediately began CST work to help him with his suck and in turn his breastfeeding. When I saw him the first time, he was in a little ball, knees to his chest and arms tucked in tight. Casey was not comfortable at all, not feeding well, and in danger of returning to the hospital if he did not gain weight. It is imperative for a little guy like Casey to continue to gain weight and thrive. His birth was traumatic; an emergency cesarean combined with all the equipment on him over those first crucial weeks caused his cranial bones to become restricted and not move correctly, which directly interfered with feeding, comfort, and function. In addition he was very constipated. Mom had tried some homeopathic remedies, Epsom salt baths, and massage, but nothing was helping. I suggested she use goat milk in addition as she built up her milk supply, and in just a matter of a few visits Casey was relaxed, lying out on the table with open hands and legs. He was feeding, alert, and having several normal bowel movements daily. His issues were simple to fix with CST, but could have been detrimental for this family had they not known what their options were to help him.

Chapter 3: First Foods & Beyond

The introduction of foods makes up the building blocks of digestive maturity. As stated before, from birth to six months, infants should survive on breast milk alone and skip rice cereal because their digestive systems are not equipped with the proper enzymes to digest food. After six months of age, infants' bodies slowly begin to make the necessary enzymes, and this continues well into the second year of life. You may increase the likelihood of future food allergies by introducing solids too soon, so it's best to take it slow. Although I look at each patient individually and their development thus far before recommending solids, a general rule of thumb would be to wait until children have teeth. The appearance of teeth is the body's way of telling you that it is producing enzymes to break down food.

Always begin introducing solids with vegetables and then move to fruits; I find that some children refuse vegetables once fruits are introduced, so get through your list of vegetables before proceeding to the sweets. They love the sweet taste of fruit, so once introduced, make sure you are giving two parts veggies to one part fruit. At any age, it is best not to eat fruits within a half hour of eating any other foods since they digest quickly and will not allow other food to be properly taken in and utilized as nourishment. Each food needs to be introduced slowly, one at a time.

When beginning solid foods, it's best to try a different food each week, adding one at a time to look for reactions. Some common reactions include changes in appetite, behavior, bowel movements, and sleep. I refer to them as the 4 Red Flags, which are discussed in depth in chapter 7.

There are so many options when starting solids, and some of my favorites are carrots, squash, zucchini, and sweet potatoes. It takes time for the body to become familiar with a new food. Although this is an exciting time as a parent, please be cautious as your child's digestive system is in development and overload is a factor. If you use small amounts to introduce one food per week, you and your infant will be well on your way.

For example:

- **Week one:** Introduce squash and feed only that solid for one week, looking for reactions (see "four red flags" in Chapter 7). If no reaction occurs, then add another food the second week.
- **Week two:** Serve squash and introduce carrots, looking for a reaction to carrots.
- **Week three and beyond:** Follow the same steps as you add a new food every week. If you see or sense a reaction, then remove that food immediately and take note of it. Take a break from introducing new foods until the reaction your child had has cleared up, so you can tell going forward what your child is reacting to as you add new foods.

Parents often ask me about giving juice to their infants. Vegetable juices, especially freshly juiced carrots, are wonderful starter foods for your baby. Juicing has become increasingly popular with many recipe options available. It is a great way to get fresh, raw greens into your family's diet. Make sure you cut the juice with distilled water or water purified by reverse osmosis.

Avoid using bottled water, which may contain chlorine or fluoride; both are known toxins.

Another great natural drink option for children is to pour a whole bag of frozen organic fruit into a pitcher of water and refrigerate it overnight. The fruit will infuse flavor into the water, making it more enjoyable for your child to drink and giving you a juice alternative.

If you choose to buy juice from the store, ensure that it is organic, not from concentrate, and free of high fructose corn syrup. It is best to dilute the juice: one-third juice, two-thirds water. Remember that a high content of natural sugar (fructose) may be too much and can overload your child's system. Store-bought concentrated juices have higher sugar content and are a known cause of yeast infections in children. As with all first foods, introduce fruit juices with caution, and follow the same rules by introducing one type of juice at a time. After all, juice is food in a liquid form and needs to be watched just the same.

As you start on the journey of new foods, don't buy baby food in a jar—the equivalent of fast food. Jarred baby food, even organic, is mostly water with high contents of sugar and salt. You can save money by pureeing the fresh veggies you have and feeding them for your child. I also know moms who pour the puree into ice trays and freeze them to have food on the go when they need it. I love that trick!

On the journey through solid foods, many parents wonder when to introduce animal sources of protein. Proteins help make up the building blocks of the body and are needed for growth, and there are many protein sources for your child. Some early protein options include cooked chickpeas or adzuki beans; they are easy to eat and make great finger foods. You can also use almond butter, cashew butter, and sesame butter, which are great sources of protein too. Just make sure your child doesn't have nut allergies ahead of time. It is recommended to hold off on meat protein until one year, but even then, move very slowly. Unlike beans, meat protein takes days for the body to digest and could be too much for a developing digestive system. When you do begin to introduce meat, stick to lean meats, like turkey and chicken, and buy organic meats free of antibiotics and hormones. With seafood, stick to white fish and avoid shellfish due to the high possibility of allergens.

As children move into toddlerhood and beyond, many come into my office with a list of foods they love, and it's common for their favorites to be white and processed. They love cheese, yogurt, cereal, pasta, chicken nuggets, pizza, and crackers. These foods may contain white flour that goes through a bleaching process, removing all its nutrients. Pastas are mostly made from processed wheat flour and tend to clog the bowels, causing gas, constipation, bloating, and digestive discomfort. When considering traditional grains, I find it best to avoid them until after the age of two. The immune system is still developing, and it's best to ensure their bodies can handle the insult when their systems are ready.

Gluten-free grains, including quinoa and tapioca, can be introduced earlier than two years if tolerated. In my experience, I have seen an abundant rise in the amount of children sensitive to gluten, the protein found in wheat, oats, barley, and rye, to name a few. For those children who are sensitive to it, this can be very irritating to the digestive system and will create larger issues with food assimilation, growth, and inflammation. If you choose gluten-free grains, I still suggest waiting until after age two, ensuring proper digestive and pancreatic enzymes for carbohydrate breakdown. It is important to note that even gluten-free grains can be binding and hard to break down for some young children; if you see signs of this, then remove the food source and wait to reintroduce grains.

Americans are programmed to give milk (mammalian) to their children once they are weaned. As part of the processed food diet, many kids love milk, yogurt, and cheese, all of which contain casein. Along with gluten, casein can also be extremely irritating to the digestive tract. Casein is the protein found in all dairies and is best avoided until after eighteen months, if consumed at all. Casein should be avoided altogether if either parent or any siblings have an allergy or sensitivity to casein. Many infants will have trouble with dairy from the start, so you might already know this is an irritant. All dairy, including cheese and yogurt, are mucus producing, yielding allergic reactions and bowel issues in many cases. In my practice, the parents that remove gluten and casein from their children's diets report increased bowel movements, healthy weight, improved sleep, normal appetite, and good behavior. Parents who worry about calcium intake can give more leafy greens, broccoli, and sesame butter as a supplement.

Here is a small list of first food do's and don'ts that were covered in this chapter:

Do's
Squash

Carrots

Zucchini

Cooked chickpeas

Sweet potatoes

Spinach

Peas

Peaches

Pears

Melons

Don'ts

Gluten (grain protein)

Casein (dairy protein)

Berries (high probability of allergy)

Fruit juice

Rice cereal

Grains (wait until age two)

Bottled water

Peanut butter (high probability of allergy)

Sugar

Honey (avoid before twelve months)

Jarred baby food (fast food for infants)

Shellfish (high probability of allergy)

Eggs (high probability of allergy)

Aspartame (artificial sugar; see Chapter 14 for detailed information)

Citrus fruit (may be hard on the stomach)

Chapter 4: Food Allergies

One of the most common irritants for children is food, contributing to massive amounts of ongoing inflammation. Most adults know if they have allergies, whether they are to food or to the environment. What are less well-known are food sensitivities; this is not the same as a food allergy. Pediatricians commonly do a conventional food allergy test, which specifically looks at the IgE immunoglobins. The foods tested can produce a histamine release within the body and are the ones people think of as classic food allergies, such as eggs and peanuts. Referred to as type 1 food allergies, these are uncommon, affecting approximately 2–5% of the population, mostly children.

However, a food sensitivity test measures IgG immunoglobins, the most common, and looks at long-term exposure to a specific food. IgG food allergies are a delayed onset food allergy, considered type 3 reactions, and 40–60% of the population has reported having a delayed food allergy. Unlike IgE food reactions, an IgG food reaction will not always give obvious signs like a rash or hay fever. The signs of IgG sensitivity range and are usually subtle in children.

Immunoglobin chart:

Immunoglobin	% of Population	Function	Affect
IgE	2–5	Traditional allergies "Classic allergy to food"	Release histamine with exposure. Reaction takes minutes to hours.
IgG	40–60	Long-term exposure "Sensitivity to food"	Delayed onset food allergy. Reaction takes hours to days.
IgM	Varies	Recent acute exposure aka "Oral tolerance"	Immune response
IgA	Varies	Past exposure	Immune response

Building Blocks: Here is a sample list of the most common symptoms seen with IgG food sensitivities.

Abdominal pain	Aches and pains
Acne	ADHD
Aggression	Anxiety
Arthritis	Asthma
Autism	Bloating
Celiac Disease	Chronic fatigue
Chronic infections	Constipation
Depression	Dizziness
Ear infections	Eczema
Enuresis (bed wetting)	Fibromyalgia
GI issues	Hyperactivity
Irritable bowel syndrome	Itching
Lethargy	Loss of appetite
Migraine	Nausea
Sinus infections	Stomach cramps
Weight gain/loss	Wheezing

IgG immunoglobins can cross the placenta, and they provide immunity to the growing fetus throughout pregnancy and the first six months of development. For this reason, many breastfeeding mothers notice changes in their infants' stool and overall comfort depending on what they are themselves ingesting. I always ask a mom to refrain from the foods she is sensitive to, especially during pregnancy and breastfeeding, due to these inflammatory processes. It is not uncommon for a child's food sensitivities to be closely related to those of their mother.

Chances are you have worked with your hands repetitively at some point, whether for work or sports, and developed calluses. This is because the repeated use of one's hands causes the skin to react to being aggravated on a regular basis. Similar reactions can be seen with the repeated ingestion of irritating foods, causing damage to the digestive system and activation of the immune response over and over again. The recurring inflammation can wreak havoc on a child's developing digestive system and brain. If you take into account that roughly 70% of the immune system is found in the gut, it's clear why food can be a contributing cause of inflammation. The digestive tract— comprised of the mouth, esophagus, stomach, small and large intestines, and anus—connect the gut and the brain. So when the gut is inflamed, it naturally works its way up into the neurological system, contributing to and in some cases creating the developmental delays seen in children.

As you can see, we have already found a way to avoid possible developmental delays: by knowing which foods irritate our bodies. I am a huge advocate of both IgE and IgG blood testing. This knowledge enables a mother to know what to eat during her pregnancy, thereby eliminating a potential cause of undue inflammation for her and the baby. If you have a child and are wondering about these sensitivities, then ask your physician to order testing; there are even finger-prick tests available to take at home.

Most physicians will order an IgE test for the top eight allergens, and most likely they will all be negative. A smaller portion of physicians will order the IgG testing for food sensitivities. It is important to note that if your child is under the age of two, allergy testing can be inconclusive, so the mom can be tested and use her results to plan the proper introduction of foods. If you have a problem getting these tests ordered, I suggest you find a biomedical, integrative, or functional medicine doctor. These specialists are more in tune with the need for these tests and will also help you understand and implement the results.

Dr. Brooks Tip:
Most insurance companies will not pay or reimburse for a finger prick blood test, but are likely to cover a full blood draw done at a local lab or at the doctor's office.

Many parents do not know to ask for IgG testing but have had IgE testing done to find out all is normal, so they naturally think that their child has no issues with food. Despite negative allergy test results, many parents still try dietary changes because they have read that a gluten-free diet can help their child, but they do so without understanding how this affects the body. An allergy (IgE) and sensitivity (IgG) are different. Some people experience distress when eating gluten products and show improvements when these are taken out of the diet. The reactions one can have range from changes in behavior, sleep, and appetite to weight loss/gain and abnormal bowel movements. The sensitivities get worse with time and are many times dependent on the sources. Not every gluten item will give the same symptom, some more than others. The medical implications of gluten sensitivity over time include significant amounts of inflammation in the small intestine, and common symptoms seen with gluten intolerance resemble gastrointestinal symptoms such as bloating, gas, abnormal bowels, nausea, seizures, anemia, fatigue, headaches, and body pain. Many gluten-sensitive children will also have nutrient deficiencies, and this always contributes to the problem. Most people get confused about the differences between an allergy, celiac disease, and non-celiac gluten intolerance. This can be very confusing, and many mistakenly treat them equally. The difference matters when dealing with long-term management and health.

Food allergies affect almost 11 million people living in the US, and IgE-mediated allergies are the most commonly known. IgE (immunoglobin E) is an antibody, a type of protein that works against a specific food. There are eight top food allergies the FDA identifies: wheat, eggs, soy, milk, peanuts, tree nuts, shellfish, and fish. Some children will outgrow their allergies and often do not receive proper nutritional interventions.

Another gluten-related condition is celiac, a digestive disease that results in damage to the small intestine; it is genetically inherited and chronic, meaning it cannot be outgrown like allergies. When those with celiac ingest gluten, their bodies have an immune response, making this an autoimmune disease. The response to gluten damages the small intestine and causes nutrients to pass through the digestive tract without being absorbed, leading to malnourishment, failure to thrive (defined in Chapter 7), and distress within the digestive system. Some common symptoms seen with celiac disease resemble gastrointestinal symptoms such as bloating, gas, abnormal bowels, nausea, seizures, anemia, fatigue, skin irritation, memory problems, headaches, and body pain. To diagnose celiac, your doctor will start with blood work, and if these tests are positive, a bowel biopsy can be performed for a definitive diagnosis. Many parents choose not to do a biopsy and simply opt to refrain from gluten items. There is no "cure" for celiac per se, but much can be done to help beyond eliminating gluten from the diet. Most people with celiac disease also have other health issues and concerns that are related to their diagnosis, and these related problems need to be addressed to truly get relief.

Non-celiac gluten intolerance/sensitivity is becoming more common. Some say there is no IgE allergy to gluten, that the wheat allergy is a reaction to another component and not to gluten itself. Others argue that wheat allergies are an actual IgE response to gluten, and as always with these situations, the debates continue. What can be definitively said is that a true IgE allergic reaction is NOT celiac disease; this is a common misnomer among patients. The common symptoms seen with food intolerance are diarrhea, stomach pain, nausea, and vomiting.

To rule out gluten sensitivity, it's best to ask your physician for an IgG food allergy test, which is designed to look at sensitivities to gluten as well as many other foods. In my private practice, I always test children for both types of immunoglobins, IgE and IgG. Most people do not have a classic allergy but do suffer with sensitivities, making certain foods reactive within their body. Reactions to food include developmental delays, pain, inattention, learning disabilities, eczema, sensory processing issues, bowel issues, sleep trouble, poor growth, and picky eating.

Building Blocks

- IgE Allergy:
  - o Reaction: Proteins or chemicals in food yield an immune reaction.
  - o Reaction Time: Immediate, minutes to hours

- Celiac Disease:
  - o Reaction: Proteins (Gliadin and Glutenins) yield an immune reaction.
  - o Reaction Time: Delayed, approx. 30 minutes to 24 hours

- Food Sensitivity:
  - o Reaction: Proteins, carbohydrates, or other chemicals in the food cause a reaction, but not an immune reaction.
  - o Reaction Time: Slow and delayed, several hours to days

Diagnosing the difference between an intolerance and celiac disease requires proper testing with your physician. Either way, there are things that can be done nutritionally to support the body and, in some cases, eliminate a food allergy. If you suspect you or your child have an allergy, make an appointment with your physician.

Building Blocks:

Sometimes parents come to me with nightmare stories about working with their child's doctor. One particular mom sought me out after doing much research and asking for testing from her pediatrician. Upon getting the results, she was told all was normal, but she didn't believe it. Her two sons were suffering from eczema, headaches, stomachaches, and inattention. In obvious confusion, she came to me. I looked over the testing and saw some red flags, so I did additional blood work. To nobody's surprise, I found out her eldest son Ben had celiac disease, and his previous doctor had run the wrong test to determine it. Her youngest son had IgG food sensitivities to gluten along with several other foods. The most important part of restoring health in a child is figuring out what is wrong, the underlying cause of the presenting problems, and that requires proper tests. Once I narrowed things down, the parents and I got their diet back on track, and today both boys are perfectly healthy and happy. This mom didn't give up; she got another opinion and perhaps saved her children from a lifetime of pain and suffering.

Chapter 5:
The Origin of Developmental Delays

Every parent asks me how the delay their child is experiencing came to be, and each situation requires a different answer. The delay could look like ADD, ADHD, pervasive developmental disorder (PDD), autism, sensory processing disorder (SPD), Asperger's, or oppositional defiance disorder, to name a few. In some cases the delay is a symptom with no diagnosis. Having a diagnosis is not necessary to go forward with treatment, because your goal should be to get to the root of what is causing the symptoms and treat your child as a whole, not just address the disorder. No matter how small or large the delay may be, there is always an underlying reason.

I have touched a bit on genetic factors and also introduction of food, two strong and compelling ways children develop abnormally. One must also account for environmental factors of delays, such as chemicals, vaccinations, food sources, geographic area, activities, and daily habits. Most parents take their children to a pediatrician for regular check-ups, and that is when children are screened for developmental milestones. If at any point doctors have reason to be concerned, they will refer parents to a developmental pediatrician for a thorough evaluation. Evaluations can also be performed by school districts, psychiatrists, and early childhood programs.

When "no" means "yes"

Our society is programmed to follow doctors' orders and not question their medical expertise. When a parent has a concern about development, in many instances the doctor will say, "Your child will catch up," or, "They will outgrow it." And, my favorite, "He is a boy. They're just slower." These responses can be extremely frustrating for a family. So, if you are told, "don't worry about it," and still doubt your doctor, then get another opinion from a doctor who specializes in special needs or developmental delays. This is imperative since treatment is generally easier when kids are younger and results can be realized more quickly. The longer you wait, the worse your child's delays could get. It's always better to know if something is going wrong, because once a problem is identified, you can get to work on healing. As a parent, you may have lingering concerns even though your child's doctor tells you that everything appears to be fine. My advice is to quench your curiosity and dig as deep as you need to until you are satisfied with the answer.

Building Blocks:

I have seen so many families over the years that were told over and over that all was fine, but they had a feeling something was really wrong. In many cases, they turned out to be right. Nathan's family came to me absolutely at their wits' end; their son was always ill with no medical explanation. He had been hospitalized several times, and labs never showed anything significant. Not to mention he had seen dozens of specialists, all of whom told his parents there was nothing to be concerned about. The family came to me, and I began to work with them on Nathan's diet, nutrition, sensory processing, constipation, fatigue, and failure to thrive.

I suspected Lyme disease. The parents were focused on his poor immune system and were not worried about any of his other symptoms, so it was imperative for me to educate them on how all these individual symptoms together pointed to him being immune compromised. I ran some of my usual tests and found rampant Candida, dysbiotic bacteria, Lyme, celiac, and early signs of irritable bowel from the years of inflammation. You can imagine how scary yet comforting this was for the family. For once they were able to confirm their suspicions that he was ill, and there was hope for him to recover and feel great.

I worked first on his Candida, dysbiotic bacteria, Lyme, and dietary changes, which seemed to clear up his lack of appetite and fatigue. He began to gain weight for once, and his bowel movements were normal. The family worked with an occupational and speech therapist for his sensory processing issues, and we continued to support his immune system in any way we could. Nathan will be under care for most of his life, as will most children this ill. As they grow, their bodies and symptoms change, and having someone to call and keep track of their health keeps them from going back to that place of hopelessness. Treatment can take time, and quality matters when you have a child like Nathan. His body did not follow the textbook definitions of his ailments, nor were any of his issues obvious. In conjunction with extensive biomedical care, I did regular chiropractic adjustments. I am happy to report that after ten months of hard work with him and his amazing parents, Nathan is happy and healthy. He had an amazing summer of progress in his speech, in addition to his improved diet, weight, and sensory function.

Chapter 6:
Gut Relation to Developmental Delays

Developmental delays of all types are merely labels of a disease process, but they do not serve to tell the story about how they came into existence— only that there is a resulting problem. The allopathic, or traditional, world of medicine treats developmental delays as more psychiatric or genetic in nature, meaning they can only be helped by prescribing medications. You can find an endless line of parents who will attest to the fact that medications didn't treat their children's conditions. Any functional or biomedical doctor will tell you that the root cause of most delays starts in the gut at some point in development, and therefore they concentrate on healing the gut to improve development or reverse a given diagnosis. Three of the most common underlying reasons for developmental delays are dysbiosis, leaky gut, and Candida.

Dysbiosis

Dysbiosis is the medical term used to describe an imbalance within the digestive tract. This imbalance can also occur on other mucous membranes but is most prominent in the digestive system. As explained before, a large majority of the immune system is housed in the gut, and the colonies of microbes that live there need to stay in balance to keep the environment happy and healthy. The good bacteria protect the body from pathogenic, or bad, microbes and keep one another in balance so that no specific colony will be in abundance. This delicate balance is often disrupted by overgrowths and can affect one or more colonies, causing damage and creating chaos in the digestive tract.

There are many causes of dysbiosis. Some children never acquire good bacteria colonies to begin with, and this may be due to not being breastfed or the mother not having an abundant amount of good bacteria to pass along during breastfeeding. Many times the use of antibiotics is the vehicle by which dysbiosis begins in children. With antibiotics, the medication is not smart enough to know what to kill, good vs. bad bacteria, so it wipes out the whole colony to make sure the infection is eliminated. This will get rid of the infection, but doesn't help the gut restore its healthy flora.

The use of pre- and probiotics helps to restore normal flora and in turn regains colony balance to the gut, keeping the immune system happy. It is imperative to use these for several months and to change the types of probiotics being given and thus rotate the cultures being restored. The probiotics bought at the store are typically the same strain, but your doctor can order higher and more diverse cultures for you and can also test to make sure balance has been restored. It is also important to note that consuming food sources containing probiotics, such as yogurts, is not enough to repopulate colonies of good bacteria and will not do what is necessary for restoration.

When a bacteria imbalance goes untreated for long enough, the pathogenic microbes take over the gut, and disease can manifest. All bacteria colonies excrete waste products; this is normal (all living things produce waste), and the body can typically handle it without problems. As these pathogenic colonies take over, the waste increases and begins to burden the body, spurring on the symptoms of dysbiosis:

- Fatigue
- Constipation and/or diarrhea
- Reflux
- Bloating
- Gas
- Undigested food in stool
- Poor behavior
- Problems with appetite/eating

If left untreated or not adequately treated, this simple imbalance, which could have been corrected, manifests into leaky gut.

Leaky Gut

The term leaky gut is used to describe the intestinal permeability of one's gut. The intestines have a barrier that allows only properly digested foods to pass through and enter the bloodstream. The small spaces in between the cells are called tight junctions; they are sealed closed to undigested food. When the lining becomes irritated, the tight junctions loosen, becoming hyperpermeable or "leaky" and allowing large food molecules to pass through undigested. These large molecules activate the immune response because they are unwanted and not properly broken down. Over time these leaky junctions become more hyperpermeable, allowing pathogenic bacteria, viruses, parasites, and toxins into the bloodstream. Yet again the immune system is triggered, and antibodies are discharged into the system to fight the intruders. The fight creates inflammation and irritates the entire body. Some symptoms you may see in your child include:

- Insomnia
- Food allergies
- Abdominal pain
- Gluten sensitivity or intolerance
- Malnutrition
- Anxiety
- Fatigue
- Constipation and/or diarrhea
- Reflux
- Bloating
- Gas
- Undigested food in stool
- Poor behavior
- Problems with appetite/eating

This inflammation has been associated with celiac, Crohn's disease, allergies, autism spectrum disorders (ASD), ulcerative colitis, psoriasis, irritable bowel, and autoimmune disease. Leaky gut can be caused by chronic stress to the body, intestinal infections, candidiasis (yeast infection), parasites, untreated dysbiosis, and/or poor diet. Until you can get to your doctor for proper testing and treatment, it is best to avoid the following:

- Sugar, which feeds yeast
- Processed foods, which may cause more irritation
- Dairy, which contributes to constipation and may feed yeast
- Fermented products, which feed yeast
- Gluten, an inflammatory food source

This is not to be taken lightly. When a child shows early signs of dysbiosis, developmental delays may be a result if left untreated.

The Yeast Connection

Many kids come into my practice with a laundry list of symptoms, and just as many parents are surprised to find out that it's all due to pathogenic systemic yeast (AKA systemic Candida) growing in their child's digestive system. You can imagine many parents are angry, and they ask, "Why was this not considered by our family doctor or pediatrician?" Let me first defend the family doctors: They often don't know that this underlying issue exists, nor are they taught to look for or treat this epidemic. Many practicing physicians have long since graduated from medical school, and unless they keep current with functional medicine (a relatively new and small branch of the large field of medicine), they wouldn't know about the many effects of Candida. Eventually parents find their way to someone who addresses the biomedical or functional medicine aspects of children's health, and POOF!—the culprit is found.

Delayed and/or special needs children are the hardest hit by yeast because they have weakened immune systems and abnormal detoxification systems that are fragile. Many have had several of rounds of antibiotics to treat their recurring infections. Please note that Candida can be seen in children who have never had antibiotics; this is simply the most common source. There are many reasons a child may have yeast, including:

- Antibiotics
- Concentrated juices high in sugar
- Undigested iron (as discussed in Chapter 2)
- Unbalanced flora (not enough, or imbalanced, good bacteria)

The most common way a child gets yeast is by antibiotic use. Since antibiotics can't differentiate between bacteria type, they go into the system and eliminate all the good bacteria with the bad, leaving an imbalance in the gut. The yeast takes advantage of this blow to the system, populating and multiplying in the digestive tract. The growth of yeast itself is slow in most cases and can take years to become symptomatic. In many cases when looking at a child's health history in infancy, symptom progression, and medication use, I can see that they have had an overgrowth of yeast for most of their life. Unfortunately, this is a common occurrence, so much so that I see it in approximately 80% of kids tested.

The symptoms range by age, exposure, and underlying medical issues. Symptoms may include bloating, gas, delayed speech, OCD, unresolved bedwetting, pain behaviors (head banging, hitting themselves), decreased attention, cognitive impairment, constipation, foul smelling stool, inappropriate laughter, eczema, intermittent aggression, and poor behavior that is unexplained. With aggression, many parents seek answers when they receive multiple complaints from school or have an inability to control their child at home.

If your child is experiencing any of the symptoms mentioned above, then it's best to consult with someone immediately to see if testing is necessary. Your child can have only one of those symptoms and have yeast. The fact is that yeast doesn't go away on its own; it just grows and gets worse.

In few cases the use of natural anti-fungal treatments has been effective in complete elimination of yeast. The natural agents slow the yeast growth down, and with this, parents may even see a short period of symptom reversal. However, parents need to seek care with a biomedical or functional medicine doctor for this treatment, because these professionals are trained in how to deal with specific issues pertaining to the digestive system, including yeast. The doctor will perform stool and urine testing to determine if pathogenic (bad) yeast is present, and this will also reveal other details necessary for treatment. Not every stool test is the same, so your pediatrician or GI specialist may not order the correct type. Biomedical/

functional medicine doctors use specific tests for Candida to ensure they collect the proper information needed for successful treatment. Seeing a doctor who's experienced with dysbiosis and Candida will ensure that you don't waste time or money.

Building Blocks:

Candida can present in any case and sometimes in those where it's least expected. A girl named Sammy, age one, came to me with constipation and chronic ear infections. She had only had one round of antibiotics but seemed to have GI symptoms worth worrying about, so I tested her stool and urine, which revealed Candida. Many people think it takes several rounds of antibiotics to begin Candida growth, but in Sammy's case, she never had enough beneficial bacteria or proper balance in her gut. With an antibiotic introduced to an already delicate situation, as if they were waiting for the opportunity to strike, dysbiosis and candidiasis occurred. This is a prime example of how one round of antibiotics can do damage. Parents must be aware, like Sammy's mom, and seek help at the first signs. She did great through treatment and is now healthy.

There are many things that doctors need to clear up when yeast is found, because like I said before, it doesn't travel alone. When yeast is present, I have found it best to attack it from a variety of ways with initial treatment lasting for approximately four months. The test results will outline proper medications for the elimination of the specific yeast that tested positive or reactive. The variety and length of treatment help to eliminate all the subtypes of yeast that present.

The best way to keep yeast at bay long-term is to make sure you test and treat the yeast effectively, heal the digestive system, and keep in line with any dietary recommendations that were made by your child's doctor. Probiotics can be helpful when using quality products properly, but remember that this alone does not rid the body of yeast. Lastly, find a way to keep your child healthy throughout the year to avoid the use of antibiotics that may spawn a new growth of yeast. I work diligently with families to ensure each child is healthy in all respects, because the last thing parents want is to have to give their child antibiotics again and treat yeast for another four months.

There is always a time and place for medicinal use, but I have found that monthly visits to a chiropractor for adjustments, coupled with supplementation to keep the immune system at its best, have made for much success in my practice. Also, be aware that not all prescriptions are the same. In my experience very few pediatricians understand systemic yeast, particularly since it's only recently come under close inspection, so it's important that you and your doctor educate your pediatrician at every corner. Don't be afraid to tell them how great your kid is doing when you see the results—it brings power to the treatment and education to the forefront.

Building Blocks:

One of the more severe cases I have come across had to do with the behaviors exhibited by David, an eight-year-old with autism and Down syndrome. His mother decided to come alone for the first visit, which is rare in my office, so I knew she had things to tell me that she did not want him to hear. David was struggling with sleep, attention, bowel movements, bloating, gas, aggressive and impulsive behaviors, eczema, and the worst of all, his behavior. David had screaming fits, and these weren't any old tantrums. He was pounding his fists on counters, biting himself, and physically lashing out at his parents. The last straw for his mother was when she caught him smearing feces on a bathroom wall; she was mortified and also very concerned. All his doctors chalked his behavior up to being autistic and having Down's, but his mom knew better. David hadn't always been like this, so she knew there must be something really wrong.

The smearing of feces is not all that uncommon, but is something parents often choose not to tell their child's doctor. This behavior is a sign of a child's massive discomfort and is perhaps a way for them to communicate their pain. I explained to Mom that this incident was okay and that I simply had to figure out what was causing him so much pain.

It was obvious he had some major digestive issues as he had all the classic signs. I tested him and found Candida. I also changed his diet and used CST (which he really loved) to help with his sleep and attention. I worked with his endocrinologist to get his thyroid meds under control and saw a real change in his labs when things were modified. David was stubborn in most instances, but always loved to come see me. Because he knew how much better he would feel once he left, he did amazingly in my office. Today, David is happy and healthy, and I get to see him once a month for his chiropractic adjustment and CST appointment, which help him maintain his alignment and mood. He is no longer combative, but is now a joy to have around.

I see and talk with parents, whether in my office or in public, and they often say, "We are going to wait to see what happens for a while." This is playing with fire. It can't be said enough: Yeast doesn't go away. Instead it grows, gets much worse, takes over the digestive system, and causes immense inflammation that can impair children neurologically. This inflammation is seen in developmental delays of all kinds. When treated, many parents see a regression in symptoms within the first week, and in the long-term, they see additional strides made in therapy and at school. You have nothing to lose by testing and everything to improve upon if something is found.

Chapter 7: Four Red Flags

During the discussion of first foods in Chapter 3, I touched upon the fact that parents need to be looking for signs and/or reactions when introducing foods. The Four Red Flags are signs and/or reactions that apply in all aspects of development, and they can be used to determine when a child needs medical attention or when to look more closely at a problem. To treat the body as a whole, *all* aspects of the body must be considered. The four things parents need to look at are appetite, behavior, bowel movements, and sleep, because together they make up the basic functioning of the body as a whole. These are the four fundamental keys to good health, and they tell doctors everything they need to know when deciding on treatment for a child.

Developmentally delayed children likely have issues in all four of these areas, yet even one red flag can cause severe issues. Do not ignore the symptoms just because they may not seem that bad now, or because your child only seems mildly affected—ignoring it today breeds more pain later. It's best to get care and guidance as soon as possible. You may in fact save your child from a developmental delay by watching for the Four Red Flags.

Four Red Flags
1. Appetite
2. Behavior
3. Bowel movements
4. Sleep

The following sections will detail each of the red flags to help you get familiar with what to look for, and examples are provided to help you understand the importance of these four things to the overall functioning and development of your child.

Appetite

Looking at a child's appetite is important in determining growth, energy levels, and overall health. Many times parents don't seek help for this, chalking it up to normal picky eating. I have news for you: There is no such thing as a normal picky eater. My goal here is to keep you from seeing a decline in growth before getting some help. When discussing a child's appetite, you must consider the amount they eat, how often they eat, and what they eat. Some of the more pronounced issues with appetite come when looking at picky eaters and those who fail to thrive.

Many times, children will not complain about stomachaches or indigestion. Why? They may have felt like this their entire life, so a stomachache becomes normal. Because they don't know what life is like without stomach pain or nausea, it doesn't seem unusual to them. Additionally, many children on the autism spectrum have very high pain thresholds. To give you an idea, I have seen children with broken bones and burst eardrums who never complained to their parents about pain. Just because a child does not complain does not mean there isn't cause for concern.

I would like to break appetite down by each instance that you may be facing to clarify what you will want to look for in your child. There are children who will eat very small portions or not eat often enough, and this may not seem like an issue until an adult sees the changes in their weight or overall appearance when undressed. I find many times that these children in particular have reflux, food allergies/sensitivities, chronic digestive inflammation, and/or dysbiosis (imbalance in the gut flora). All under-eaters have trouble digesting foods, but the types of foods depend on what else is happening in their digestive system. A simple stool and urine test can determine what is happening inside their digestive tract, and blood work can determine deficiencies and imbalances in their system. If you put together a plan to heal the gut and feed the deficiencies, you will see an increase in appetite and therefore an increase in amount of food eaten. Children are very smart and intuitively know what bothers them from infancy, so if your child refuses certain foods, take that as a possible food allergy or sensitivity and investigate it further with your biomedical doctor to determine if it is an important factor.

Building Blocks

This past year Ingrid, a teenage girl, and her mom came in to see me. The family ate all homemade, organic, vegan food and kept a chemical-free home, but Ingrid seemed distant and almost depressed. She saw the family chiropractor regularly for adjustments and, to anyone looking in, seemed ultra-healthy; yet Ingrid was not thriving, not gaining weight, and was in pain. Ingrid had no appetite and was unable to eat but very small portions without having abdominal discomfort. Her mother would space out her meals to try to help keep the stomach pain at bay, but it simply was not working, and her health was deteriorating.

Her mother was also thin, so Ingrid's weight was of no major concern until one day her mom saw her undressing and could see her bones. This was her red flag to get help. I took the necessary steps and tested her stool, urine, and blood. I had them keep a food diary and note the intensity of her stomachaches on a scale so her mom and I could try to see a pattern with foods. After about two weeks of tracking her diet, I could see some patterns emerging. I eliminated foods that I suspected were irritating to her and added digestive support to help her break down her food correctly. Her stomach pains began to lessen a bit. I then focused on the lab results and treated the underlying GI issues she presented with, which yielded great results in her energy, weight gain, and mood. To cap it all off, I did some food allergy testing and identified some of the suspected culprits along with additional foods she and Mom were going to work through via an elimination diet.

It is amazing how much a child suffers socially and emotionally when they do not feel well. Food can be a major source of pain. By learning what she should eat and what to avoid, Ingrid's life was changed in a positive way. In the time I saw Ingrid, I was able to see her come out of a fog. She even made a drawing for me, which hangs proudly in our office to remind me of her healing and journey. I had an opportunity to heal, empower, and educate her about the foods her body was irritated by, thus making a happier and healthier teenager who will continue to flourish.

The picky eaters are perhaps my favorite cases because it's so fun to see them go from eating five foods to eating unthinkable things that shock their parents. I have parents swear their children will never eat well, but with proper treatment, these kids blossom into curious little foodies. As discussed earlier, many of these children feel awful and hide their pain, and picky eaters have it the worst. Everyone remembers being told or telling their own child, "Don't touch the stove—it's hot!" But what happens? They touch it and learn that, not only were you right, but they don't want to go anywhere near that stove again. Well this is how introduction to foods goes with children too.

Children's digestive problems begin in infancy most of the time, and as food is introduced, they begin to realize which foods harm or hurt them and which ones do not. So, being wise, they decide that if the mashed potatoes made them feel upset, then they should avoid them, much like the hot stove, and add mashed potatoes to the list of things they don't like. In many cases this seems okay. Not everyone can like everything, right? That may be the case, but as children grow, parents might begin to notice the list of things their kid doesn't like getting longer and longer until one day he's six years old and will only eat five or ten things. The list of refused foods grows as they might base refusal on color, texture, or odor. I can hear your concern from here: "My kid won't eat if I don't give her what she wants." And you're right; children might eat very poorly for the first few days when you try to change their habits. Do not try to deal with their dietary restrictions without medical supervision, because there is support available to help them digest their food, heal the gut, and take that stomachache away for good. Parents will often fail if just dealing with the food aspect of the problem, so remember that the food is the symptom—NOT the problem.

Building Blocks:

A very educated and wise mother came to me with her eight-year-old son who had been diagnosed with Asperger's and was a very picky eater. She had tried the gluten-free, casein-free diet (GFCF) years before and saw no changes in him at all. She began to get concerned as he got older and as his younger brother grew to outweigh him, and she knew he needed help. He loved gluten, and his diet was based on chicken nuggets, sandwiches, and chips. There was very little protein in his diet, and over the years she just gave up fighting his picky eating. As expected, she came to me very concerned about changes to his diet because they had always failed in the past. I reminded her that many parents fail when trying the GFCF alone because proper digestive support is needed for the treatment to be successful.

During this process, including food allergy testing, this mom learned what to feed her finicky son and what he would react to, information that's imperative to know to avoid future growth issues. I changed him back to the GFCF diet – starting with casein-free for two weeks and then adding gluten-free – and upped his protein intake. With proper digestive support, his weight improved after a few months. In addition I performed urine, stool, and blood testing and ensured he was supplemented appropriately, which also helped him to continue gaining weight. His symptoms were caused by a combo of bodily deficiencies in vitamins and other essential nutrients, plus improper digestion, all made worse by irritating foods. This is the perfect example of why it makes a difference having medical help with your child's picky eating habit. Handling the basics on your own, like this mom did, is often not enough.

The cases that give me the most heartache involve children with failure to thrive (FTT). I see very ill children in my practice, and I am so thankful they have come to me because I know their life will improve with the right treatment. There is a huge spectrum when talking about what FTT is; sometimes it is based on growth charts and other times is the sheer wasting away of a child. FTT is a medical emergency in every case and needs to be treated aggressively and immediately. The body will steal from other systems to continue functioning, so the longer you wait to begin treatment, the more the body shuts down. The FTT child typically has a long history of poor appetite and picky eating, and nothing has worked for the parents. Feeding therapy has shown some benefit, but without positive test results, the parents are left to tube feed in extreme cases. Parents facing milder cases of FTT will usually give their children whatever they want as long as they eat.

Do you see the bad pattern here? Continually feeding children whatever they want usually entails a diet comprised of foods that digestively inflame them, such as gluten and casein. Not to mention that much of the food kids choose for themselves is processed.

Building Blocks:

One patient I will never forget is Briane. She arrived in her wheelchair, fully equipped with her ventilator and g-tube. I had never seen a child that malnourished and thin. You could see all her bones, and her skin was so thin it was almost transparent. Mom was obviously doing all she could. Because Briane had been born with a genetic condition, it was a miracle she was still alive, but she surely wasn't thriving. It was imperative to run tests to see how severe the deficiencies were, and they revealed a myriad of problems. I chose to plug away at them one by one, support her body with what it needed, and not get caught up in the fact that she was being fed through a tube. At least the tube made it super easy to give her supplements because they went directly in.

It was also important to know her food allergies as many of the formulas given to FTT children are dairy-based, and in many cases like with Briane, these children have sensitivity to casein. Her mom had asked the hospital dietician if casein was a potential allergy, but they blew off her concern. The very formula prescribed by the hospital that was supposed to nourish her was actually creating inflammation, and because her body could not break the formula down, it was not helping her gain weight and thrive. Obviously, I changed the formula and began to concentrate on getting "real" food into her tube slowly over time. Briane tolerated the treatments better than expected and has progressed well.

These are the cases that bring heartache at first and joy later when the children begin to do better. Again, FTT should be seen as a symptom, not the underlying cause of what is going wrong. If you focus on the symptoms all the time, a resolution will never be found to break the cycle of what's really going on below the surface.

Take the knowledge you have learned the last few pages and ask yourself this question: Is Briane suffering digestively? Drum roll, please.... YES. I know all of you got that one right, but let's break down exactly why FTT happens.

The testing administered by the gastrointestinal (GI) specialists often comes out normal. They run tests to rule out causes for the symptoms, perhaps using a scope to see what is happening inside the body. These are great tests and do answer questions about the health of your child's gut, but what happens when they come back "normal"? Does this mean there is not a digestive issue? No, this may only mean that the problem has not gotten bad enough to show on a scope, or perhaps the portion of the GI system that's involved was not examined. A specialist is just that: someone who specializes. Therefore the GI doctor just looks at GI issues. So if the underlying cause of your child's symptoms goes beyond the GI tract, is there a chance the real problem is missed? Absolutely, and this is why it's imperative to look at all the pieces of the puzzle when treating a child.

For example, a child may exhibit inflammatory signs of Crohn's disease or inflammatory bowel disease (IBD) but the test results are normal. Every child's inflammation starts somewhere, but it may not be enough to red flag that specialist or lab technician. In my practice, I find that about 98% of the families coming in have never had the basic stool and urine tests, which pick up the less commonly known and earlier signs of inflammation and digestive distress. This is why biomedical doctors have so much success. Our toolbox contains a broader suite of instruments to determine what is needed to properly put the pieces together to see a child's picture of health. Although they can be tough to spot on a test, the broad range of issues seen in FTT is medically severe, and the causes and symptoms have to be dealt with delicately and effectively.

I hope you can see the cascade of events that start out very small and can roll into something life-threatening. The lesson to take from this is to get help regardless of how small you may think your child's health problem is. These things don't fix themselves and only breed larger medical issues with time.

Dr. Brooks Tip:
Here are some foods you can try to improve appetite:
- Cranberries
- Coconut kefir/yogurt (found in the dairy section) mixed with applesauce
- Peppermint tea

Behavior & Infants

The second red flag is behavior, which is subdivided here into infancy, adolescence, and adulthood. When parents decide to ask for help with their infant, many times it is due to abnormal behavior. In infants I see this behavior manifest as reflux or colic. But what if these issues can be traced to an underlying medical issue? In these cases, something can be done. When poor behavior is seen in infants, many times it is due to them having a hard time digesting formulas and foods (either eaten by mom or given directly). Inconsolable fussing and crying, slow weight gain, frequent vomiting/

spitting up, and trouble nursing can all be signs of birth trauma, food allergy, and food intolerance.

I have seen infants as young as three weeks get prescribed reflux medications and given the vague diagnosis of gastroesophageal reflux disease (GERD). The previous generation was told this was colic and that nothing could be done to help. Now we have a pill to give a panicked mom to make her feel better while dealing with her infant's GERD. But what about treating the infants? The truth is that these infants are uncomfortable, and reflux or colic may be the only sign of discomfort their parents get. All infants cry for a reason, and any mother knows the difference between their infant's hunger cry versus wet diaper cry. This is why colic is so frustrating for a mother—because nothing makes it better.

In my experience, less than 15% of GERD diagnoses actually have reflux, and yet this is the most common diagnosis given to newborns today. As a parent you want answers, and understandably so, but GERD isn't the right one. In 2011, *The Journal of Pediatrics* reported that infants are being overly prescribed acid-reducing medications, a small admittance in my eyes. Along with these medications, parents are instructed to thicken formula, but many report no change or worsening of symptoms. Most parents don't know that these medications are prescribed "off label." What does that mean? No pediatric studies have been performed with that medication specific to your child's diagnosis. Basically, during the initial studies the medication was approved for something other than what you are using it for, and therefore its use is not listed on the label. Physicians noticed an improvement by using it for off-label reasons, and soon enough it began to be prescribed by many others for those off-label symptoms.

In the case of GERD medications, they have been over-prescribed for off-label reasons, causing alarming side effects like headaches, constipation, vomiting, stomach pain, and rashes. I have seen these side effects too many times. The most common sign of digestive discomfort is the pulling of the knees to the chest and/or tightly closed fists. This holding of infants' bodies in a ball is just a way to tell you they hurt, even when they don't cry.

Building Blocks:

Baby Gabby was born into this world in a sea of discomfort. Mom labored for over twelve hours before having a C-section delivery, and the doctors had such a hard time getting her out that they had to use forceps because she was breeched. Gabby came out healthy, but soon after getting home, the new parents realized their new miracle baby girl would not be easy. She cried for hours and hours, would spit up one-quarter of her meal with each feeding, and seemed unhappy.

In fear something was wrong with Gabby, the parents went to their pediatrician and explained what was happening, and she was prescribed a reflux medication. The parents were so relieved to have an answer that would put an end to all the crying. Not to mention it is difficult for a new mom to bond with her baby when there is so much tension. Yet after trying the medication for a week, there was no improvement, and they decided to try something different. That is when I met Gabby. She was eight weeks old, beautiful but very uncomfortable. As I unwrapped her, I could barely get my hands under her to pick her up because she was balled up so tight, and she made these little grunting noises with each movement.

I did CST on her for her birth trauma due to Cesarean delivery and the use of forceps. A Cesarean birth does not allow proper cranial molding, which leads to restrictions in the cranial bones and will in most cases show symptoms like colic and reflux. After the first treatment, she slept for hours without crying. Gabby continued to improve with each treatment, and a few weeks later she was perfectly comfortable and feeding great. Her quick recovery was a relief to the parents, to say the least.

The best advice I can give any parent is to seek out help when you first get that gut feeling something is not right. Whatever you may be seeing or experiencing is a small indication of the underlying problem and is perhaps your first glimpse into the future. Receiving guidance along the way from someone you trust to care for your children can help your family avoid dealing with unfortunate developmental delays.

Think of it this way: When buying a new car, part of the appeal is the warranty you get with purchase. This warranty makes you feel safe and gives you a sense of peace, especially if you have ever broken down on the side of the freeway. Your doctor is your warranty, looking out for your best interests and guaranteeing help when needed. Now not all warranties are equal, which is why you need to do your homework in selecting someone who's a great fit for your family. If you have a doctor to turn to when you have concerns, and it is someone who will truly honor your child and listen to you, then you can avoid wasting all the hours spent self-researching, attending seminars, and trying expensive home treatments. So, do you have a quality warranty on your child?

It is also a good idea to find a pediatric chiropractor to see your newborn for craniosacral therapy (CST). If your child exhibits early signs of discomfort, such as colic or reflux, a pediatric chiropractor can help. This is your chance as a new parent to put your best foot forward and offer maximum health to your new gift.

Behavior & Adolescents

With poor behavior in older children, parents usually begin to get reports from teachers and are only then awakened to the wide scope of what they're dealing with. Bad behavior is hard to see sometimes; you are with your children so much and may find the school's reports hard to believe. Most parents will try discipline or reward systems only to end up with little or no success. As children grow, their bad behaviors will cover the spectrum from simply not following directions to aggression towards other kids or themselves. Again, when parents seek help, they are told to medicate their child. Not wanting to medicate but feeling there are no other options, many parents suffer in silence, searching aimlessly for information on the Internet.

There are many reasons for poor behavior. For example, when you are sick, do you feel 100%? No, you feel awful, and people are just lucky you roll out of bed and open your eyes. You might come off as being grumpy or irritable, or you could seem lazy or unenthusiastic. Well, this is how your child feels too. When their body is retaliating against them, they will act out. This behavior usually occurs in phases, and that's why it can take so long for parents to reach out to a doctor for help. It's easy to rationalize bad behaviors with real-world factors: "It's summer time, and he is getting to bed late." "Relatives are in town, and she has to share her room." "We started a new school/therapy, and he needs time to adjust." And the list goes on and on. When this behavior continues over weeks or months, even sporadically, that's a red flag that it isn't a short-term problem.

I see a lot of poor behavior as a result of systemic yeast (Candida) and other forms of dysbiosis. It is also very common for food sensitivities to affect behavior. Since trigger foods can remain in the system for several days at a time, children with food sensitivities are always reacting to triggers that are frequent in their diet and, as a result, are exhibiting that sensitivity as inattention in school or aggression at home. Many children are misdiagnosed with ADD and ADHD today when in fact it is a food sensitivity that keeps activating their system and causing the reaction.

As discussed before, a food sensitivity doesn't have to be a skin reaction, as parents are commonly trained to think. Behavior is a huge indicator of poor digestion or food intolerance. It is easy to rationalize behaviors, but going forward, that will change as you understand there is something that can be done to alleviate the underlying cause—no matter how bad your child's behavior seems.

Building Blocks:

Amy was six when her mother decided she needed to get a professional opinion on her behavior. This is a key age when parents realize via teachers, other parents, and group activities that their child's bad behavior is really too much. The final straw was when Amy had a meltdown at school and the teacher had to clear the classroom for safety reasons. This was when I met Amy. Mom reported that Amy had been aggressive since she was a toddler, often biting and scratching. As she got older and stronger, her mother began to be afraid of her, especially after Amy threatened her with a knife. Her aggression was being taken out on the entire family, and everyone was paying the price.

Amy had high anxiety, hyperactivity, and difficulty with transitions; she would also tell me it was hard for her to sleep because her mind was too busy. Most people would think she was a perfect candidate for psychotropic medication (medications used to counterbalance these behaviors, often unsuccessfully), but I saw something else after learning more about her. She had a history of recurring infections, watery stool, and pain in her stomach. Noticing that food was a huge trigger for her, I changed Amy's diet, treated her Candida, which was her primary source of aggression, and helped her with her nutritional deficiencies, sleep, anxiety, and mood modulation. I also used supplementation and CST to help Amy's behavior.

Many parents assume their child can't sit still for a prolonged period of time, and I find that these kids do the best with CST because the tension in their body is eliminated. As a result of her treatment, Amy's aggression disappeared, she had no more stomach pain, and her sleep, anxiety, and mood drastically improved. Since her behavioral problems were found to be very food-driven, she did great after changing to her custom diet.

Behavior & Special Needs Adults

As a developmentally delayed child ages into adulthood, things progress and change shape. What I mean is that their symptoms can go unnoticed or even seem to disappear; this is an illusion. Our bodies are adaptable and will do whatever is needed to keep us functioning. Children's bodies adapt to the dysfunctions and problems they face, and these may appear as another symptom that caretakers are unaware of. Symptoms may include bowel issues, stomach pain, mood swings, or problems with compliance.

Adults, especially those who are high-functioning, tend to be private about bowel habits and do not complain at all about pain, so from the outside looking in, they may appear perfectly fine until a peculiar behavior comes to the surface. Adults are an ignored part of the special needs community, and that needs to change; their access to services is limited, and many think adulthood is too late for positive change. That assumption is wrong.

Building Blocks:

Isaiah came to me at age seventeen. His mom was a dedicated mother of four children, and he was the last to leave the nest. Isaiah was "quirky," as his mom explained to me, and he had been through years of doctor appointments to help him with his Asperger's diagnosis. When he was a child, there were not many treatment options, so they were stuck in the traditional medical model of care. As he aged, she became very involved with wellness and health and sought nutritional guidance for him. In coming to me, she had high hopes that I could put any missing pieces together before he graduated from high school.

When I met with Isaiah for the first time, he had no idea why he was in my office and was a bit perturbed at his mom for bringing him. Isaiah did not complain to me about any type of symptoms or pain, but in asking questions, I could see there was more for me to investigate. I knew I wasn't going to get him to cooperate, which is totally normal. So I decided that testing would prove either way what needed to be done, and that would be something he could appreciate. Along with testing, I suggested craniosacral therapy (CST) and chiropractic adjustments. Isaiah was very OCD, very quiet, brilliant, and annoyed with others on many occasions. I thought his body could use the break that CST offers, and the therapy would give me a chance to speak with him about managing his stress.

Isaiah was a dedicated student and a perfectionist to boot. I remember having a talk with him about his Asperger's and how much of a blessing it could be in life if he knew how to properly utilize his gift. He and I engaged in conversation and exchanged ideas, which was rare for him. Conversing with Isaiah was truly one of the highlights of his treatment process for me. In treating him, I focused on his nutritional deficiencies as well as stress; he needed the full mind-body treatment. The CST and chiropractic care allowed me to help his body reduce the stress load. I also spoke with him about stress reduction techniques and, lastly, supported him nutritionally to help his body and mind function better presently and in the future. Isaiah went on to attend college, and I'm looking forward to the graduation announcement that's sure to come.

Bowel Movements

The third red flag is a topic people always shy away from, but one I always want to talk about—just ask my patients. There are many misnomers out there about how often one should poop, when to be concerned, etc. For years I have had parents tell me their child has a few poops per week and that their doctor told them this was fine. Newsflash: It's not fine, and as a matter of fact, it's terrible. It is important for the body to eliminate what it does not need, and when that process does not happen, toxic buildup can begin, leading to behavioral problems and more serious digestive issues. Infants should poop several times daily, and as kids get older, they should have at least one bowel movement per day. Is your kid a daily pooper?

Building Blocks:

Wyatt was a curious child and had the sweetest smile. I swear that when he smiled, you would give him anything he wanted. Wyatt always struggled with his immune system and with frequent pneumonia, and he had been hospitalized five times for respiratory issues in his four short years. At two he was diagnosed with pervasive developmental disorder (PDD) and celiac disease. His parents came to me for biomedical care because they were concerned; Wyatt had a habit of punching himself in the stomach, and he also struggled with bouts of diarrhea and hard stool, picky eating, hyperactivity, and sleep. I, of course, asked the parents about his bowel frequency, and they told me he had two poops daily, although consistency was abnormal. He got a clean bill of health from the GI specialist, but it nagged them that he seemed to be in pain even though "nothing was wrong." I decided to do testing to see what was happening inside his GI system and found many issues. It is imperative that a strict diet be followed for his celiac disease, particularly at this age. The family was gluten-free at the time, but he had spent three years eating gluten products before his diagnosis, which had done inflammatory damage to his system.

So, why did Wyatt hit his stomach? He, like many children, did this to try to relieve the pain, and parents can easily mistake this for a behavioral problem when in fact it is a medical issue. Via supplementation, I did an aggressive GI repair treatment on him, providing digestive support to help him break down his foods, and I focused on re-building his immune system. Wyatt also enjoyed his chiropractic adjustments and CST when he came to see me so much that he would head straight for the table.

It's amazing to see the domino effect in children when so much goes wrong from one underlying cause, but if you find the key to unlock the real trouble, you can fix it. When I treated the GI system in Wyatt, the other symptoms he had with his sleep, stool, picky eating, and self-injurious behaviors quickly went away, revealing that his digestive issues were the cause of all his other symptoms. He is now comfortable, healthy, and thriving.

The term constipation is used in many circumstances, and many people assume they are constipated any time stool is hard or hard to get out. However, constipation can be the consistency (loose or hard), frequency (how often one has a stool), and difficulty (straining, taking a long time). I label constipation as any abnormal stools with the above parameters. Being "regular," as the saying goes, has a lot to do with detoxification. Bowel movements are the major way our bodies detoxify and rid waste.

How do you feel if you go four days between poops? Awful, I bet. So, why do you think it is okay for your child? This is yet another reason why a child may misbehave, not sleep well, or have stomach pain. Not many kids like to talk about their poop; they're taught it's private. And once kids get past a certain age, usually six, they stop telling others about it or asking for help in the bathroom. So, start tracking their bowel movements and have a talk with your child about why you are asking them about their bathroom activity. You would be surprised how many kids will cooperate if you appeal to what is bothering them.

For example, if a little girl is having stomachaches, I will have this talk with her. I explain that I need her help and have a super important job for her. I need her to tell Mom when she poops so I can help her tummy feel better. I hardly ever get resistance once a child understands the goal. Never underestimate how smart and insightful your child is; kids know something's wrong and that they need help. Once you start tracking bowel movements, you may be shocked by how irregular they are, and this is an indication to seek help. If your child is still interested in stickers, you can make a chart for them to add a sticker every time they poop, with a certain number of stickers yielding a prize or special treat. This chart helps you see how often and when they have a stool so you can report back to your doctor.

Another common reason children will be constipated is because it hurts for them to go, but again, they never tell you that part. Some children have a high pain tolerance, so you may never know it is painful, but you can see the discomfort of constipation come through in other ways if you look closely at their behaviors.

Building Blocks:

Peter was a pre-teen boy with Asperger's and was very vocal about how he felt. Mom had a tough time throughout the years with Peter because the treatments available today were not available to her when he was younger. He was still struggling with potty training at twelve years old, and Mom reported that he refused to use the toilet and chose to poop in a diaper, waiting until the last moment to go. He would urinate in the toilet as needed, but when he needed to poop, he would go put on a pull-up or would wait until nighttime because he wore a diaper nightly to bed. This was frustrating for his mom because he was a bright and funny child who clearly knew what he was doing, and she just wasn't sure if he was being difficult or if there was a reason to be concerned. I have found this to be a common story in my practice; children choose a diaper because they feel more relaxed since it is slightly less painful for them when they have a stool.

Peter never complained about pain, and believe me, he complained readily about other things. But, of course, he did not want to discuss any bowel habits with me or his mom. Regardless of the embarrassment it causes, poop is always important! I know all about poop frequency, but in this case, Peter wasn't talking. I asked his mom to think of a way she could get him to report his frequency, and she came up with an idea: Every time he pooped, he got to add a marble to his jar. Peter collected marbles, so this was a cheap yet great reward for his compliance. In the meantime, I treated him with chiropractic adjustments and CST, which helped move his bowels more regularly. I also decided to test his stool, urine, and blood to see what may be causing such discomfort. After seeing his results, I changed his diet, treated Candida, and got him supplemented appropriately. After years of struggling, Peter is now fully potty trained and still such a joy to see for his regular check-ups.

Each child is different, and so are their symptoms. Bowel movements are the key to overall digestive health, and some of the more obvious signs can be seen when parents pay closer attention to bathroom habits. Signs a child may exhibit include red anal ring, itchy bottom, large volumes of stool, super stinky poop, bloating, and excessive gas. These are signs of digestive distress that need to be addressed medically.

In some cases, parents report constipation as an issue throughout their child's whole life and rely on quick fix medications such as Miralax to get them through. This is not an answer but a Band-Aid. Children do not have a deficiency in Miralax; they have an ongoing digestive issue. Please do not resort to laxatives or stool softeners without medical supervision.

Dr. Brooks Tip:

Parents report some improvement with the following changes, but this is not a substitution for seeking medical care. These can be tried in the interim as you look for a doctor:

- Increase fluids
- Increase fiber
- Decrease constipating foods, such as cow's milk, cheese, yogurt, cooked carrots, and bananas

Sleep

The importance of this last red flag is often downplayed, but it is equally vital for development. When we sleep, it is the only time our bodies repair and renew themselves. It is also when the body releases the most growth hormones, a crucial factor of proper development. The quality and quantity of sleep are equally important; truly restful sleep cannot be achieved without either. As new parents, sometimes you get lucky and have a great sleeper from day one, but (sorry to say) this is rare. As with all else, parents must look at a few things when it comes to sleep:

- Does your child fall asleep easily?
- Does your child wake during the night?
- Does your child wake rested?

All of these questions help determine if sleep is an issue. There are two parts of the nervous system that help us stay in balance: sympathetic and parasympathetic. The sympathetic is our fight or flight system, whereas the parasympathetic is in charge of resting and digesting. Ideally you want the nervous system to be in balance, meaning that the sympathetic and parasympathetic are equal. A child that is in sympathetic overload (I also refer to this as "overdrive") may have an underlying medical issue, and the system is working overtime trying to keep things together. This is a common reason why a child cannot get to sleep, because a body in overdrive has a hard time shutting down and giving itself a chance to rest.

Some children are waking throughout the night because they are in pain or are uncomfortable, but again, they probably won't tell you this. If waking is difficult and they seem tired, it's because the body is not getting into full deep sleep, many times due to stress. This stress is not the type you and I worry about as adults—it's certainly not stress from a job or mortgage. This stress is from a nervous system imbalance (discussed further as part of CST in Chapter 11). The imbalance affects the hormones, neurotransmitters, and overall functioning of one's body.

Many parents will try melatonin or natural sleep aids to help, but it is important to address the reason why your child's body cannot slow down and rest. The Band-Aid here is sleep aids, and although it is so important for children to get adequate sleep for growth, recovery, and learning, it is more important for you to figure out the root cause of the sleeping trouble so your child can truly rest.

Aside from testing with your doctor for potential underlying issues, you may also want to add craniosacral therapy (CST) to your treatment plan. For years, I have told parents that the side effect is better sleep. Many children who receive this therapy will sleep through the night for the first time in their lives, making this is a non-invasive option to add to the list (and you will surely be glad you did).

Building Blocks:

During a first appointment with a family, the parents and I always discuss the Four Red Flags, and sleep is a big part of the discussion. Many parents assume that their child sleeps fine. Unless their poor sleep keeps you up all night with them, that's an easy assumption to make. Take Cody, for example. His parents brought him to me for biomedical care for his autism. One of the first questions I asked was about sleep, and they both told me he was a good sleeper. But Cody looked absolutely exhausted to me, complete with bags under his eyes. I asked the parents to keep a closer eye on his sleeping habits.

Dad worked the night shift, so he started checking on Cody when he got in at 3 a.m., and sure enough, Cody was found playing quietly in his room. Both parents were shocked because they assumed that, since he was not disruptive, he was sleeping. They also told me he seemed to be fighting sleep almost like he was trying to stay awake. This became my biggest concern; a child with autism desperately needs this downtime, and their progress could be cut short simply because they do not sleep. I was fortunate that the parents understood my goals and were prepared to make some big changes for him.

So as not to waste any time, I started with dietary changes while waiting on test results. I used some supplements and changed their evening routine to improve his sleep. In a matter of about six weeks Cody was sleeping well through the night, and some of his autistic behaviors were gone. He began to talk a ton and was quite the social butterfly. It's amazing what sleep can do—or lack of sleep, for that matter.

I cannot stress enough how these four simple red flags could open your eyes to what may be troubling your child, and in fact, tracking these four habits could heal them. It is imperative for all you parents out there to keep a watchful eye and follow your instincts. If you feel like something is wrong, then you are probably right. You do not have to be a doctor to start the healing process for your child. Avoiding a delay or reversing one can sometimes be as simple as noticing when something is not quite right before your child's doctor realizes it. Parents should fight and advocate for what is best, and the Four Red Flags are effortless tools you can use to empower yourself.

Chapter 8: Common Developmental Delays

One in every six children is diagnosed with a developmental delay. Every child is monitored for developmental milestones, growth, and overall health. When milestones are not met, sometimes the parents are not even told. In the case of minor delays when you're told not worry, but to wait and see, I caution you not to wait. This waiting game can be a gamble on the future development of your child, so it is best to seek out another opinion and investigate further. In the worst case, the delay is not a big deal, and you can rest assured that you checked every possibility. Most times, though, families' eyes are opened to other delays that may be occurring, and treatment can begin early, which is a blessing.

There are many developmental delays that are common among children. This chapter covers autism spectrum disorders (ASD), attention deficit disorder (ADD), attention deficit hyperactivity disorder (ADHD), and sensory processing disorder (SPD). Once a diagnosis is made or a symptom is seen, your journey to healing can begin. The first step of treatment is choosing a medical team. It is imperative to find a physician and therapy team, to make sure proper lab testing is done, and to follow treatment as directed to give your child the best chance at recovery.

The autism spectrum includes pervasive developmental disorder

(PDD), autism, and Asperger's. Some doctors include sensory processing, ADD, and ADHD in the spectrum, but I will discuss these separately. ASDs occur on a spectrum because the symptoms seen in children can appear in different combinations and to different degrees, with each child being truly unique and different. This is part of the mystery in diagnostics, and for some, it's the difficulty in treatment. I want to simply define each of these delays with the common symptoms, but remember, your child hasn't exactly memorized the medical textbooks and may present slightly differently or may be undiagnosed. Having a diagnosis is not needed in order to get help.

PDD-NOS

Pervasive developmental disorder not otherwise specified (PDD-NOS) is the baby sister to autism, and it is also known as atypical autism. This diagnosis is generally given because a child is suspected of autism but has yet to meet the full criteria, perhaps due to age or simply because the diagnosing physician isn't completely convinced they have autism. Usually this label goes to children under the age of three who have communication or social delays. More times than not, children diagnosed with autism previously had a PDD-NOS label. It is imperative to see a biomedical doctor as soon as you get this diagnosis; perhaps you can avoid the "autism" diagnosis and remove the PDD one too.

There are signs of PDD-NOS that your doctor will look for:

- Difficulty using language or understanding what is being said to them
- Unusual toy play (lining up, stacking)
- Self-stimulatory behaviors aka stimming (repetitive movements, for

example flapping)

- Difficulty relating to people emotionally or socially
- Lack of appropriate eye contact
- Difficult time with transitions and changes to routine

Autism

In our current day and age, it is hard to ignore the cries of the millions of families that have a child with autism. Autism involves multifaceted symptoms of an underlying disease process that affects the immune, digestive, neurologic, and toxicological systems. Prior to 1980, finding autism was rare at 2 to 5 cases per 10,000 people. The rate is now 1 in 88 children and 1 in every 54 boys. Generations prior thought that autism was a psychiatric disorder, but the medical research has since shown that this is not the case. Parents are often told that their children's diagnosis is the result of genetics and is psychological in nature. Typical psychological manifestations in children with autism include those of PDD-NOS, plus:

- Delayed speech
- Shyness
- Delayed gross or fine motor skills
- Sensory processing issues (sound and touch sensitivity, etc.)
- Not responding to one's name
- Often unexplained changes in mood (tantrums and outbursts)
- Obsessive behaviors
- Low awareness of physical danger
- High threshold for pain
- Seizures or tics
- Focus closely on objects

The physical or medical issues children often share are rarely noted or discussed. For example, I have yet to see a child with autism who doesn't have a GI or food sensitivity/allergy issue to some degree. Your physician's job is to examine the typical physical manifestations to help in the treatment of your child as a whole. These symptoms include:

- Food allergies/sensitivities
- Eczema
- General gastrointestinal distress
- Constipation and diarrhea
- Yeast/bacterial overgrowth
- Immune system issues
- Sleep disturbances
- Bloating/gas

Despite the research and the millions of families that have recovered using biomedical interventions, many parents of ASD children are still hesitant about seeking care down this road. There are inaccuracies among parents about the definition and uses of biomedical interventions. The biomedical approach is based on scientific research that shows biological causes for autism, such as heavy metal poisoning, yeast infection, food sensitivity, and nutritional deficiencies. Biomedical intervention is based on the science that the psychological symptoms listed above are a product of the physical issues the child is experiencing. Therefore, addressing these physical issues will lead to an improvement in the psychological symptoms. This new understanding has brought recovery to many families as well as hope to those that seek an answer.

The Autism Research Institute suggests that there is a strong implication to an environmental component. If the medical community can figure out what environmental factors trigger this epidemic, we can perhaps understand how to prevent it. Children with autism have abnormal detoxification systems, and this increases their risk of damage from environmental insults. After conception, the fetus is exposed to toxins and foreign substances from the air, food eaten by the mother, and medications and vaccinations she may have received. These substances pass through Mom to the placenta and into the fetal tissue. The baby then has a weak detoxification capacity, and the toxins can accumulate rather than be excreted.

Once born, the baby continues to be introduced to toxins and chemicals, beginning with medications during delivery, or given prophylactically (e.g., giving antibiotics in case of an infection) to the baby in the hospital. In the first year, the baby comes in contact with countless new exposures, including breast milk, formula, baby food, other foods, chemicals in the air, soaps, clothes, vaccines, medications like acetaminophen or ibuprofen, and often antibiotics. Most children handle the exposures without obvious ill effects, but if a child has an abnormal immune or detoxification system, risk of injury will be much higher. As environmental toxins accumulate in the child's body, the struggling immune and/or detoxification system can no longer handle the toxins appropriately, and damage occurs.

It is important to understand that there is not one event that causes a child to become diagnosed with autism, nor is every child treated the same. Often parents can account for when the "change" in their child happened. The body is designed to handle insult and injury, but enough injury breaks it down, which is often referred to as the straw that broke the camel's back, or the tipping point of the delay. The "straw" (catalyst) may be a vaccine, illness, irritating food, or something that can't be pinpointed. My experience in treating these children has taught me time and time again that there is no singular cause; I have never found just one underlying problem.

With that said, I also want to explain that everyone is genetically predisposed to expressing things differently. Let's look at cancer, for example. Perhaps you have a long family history of cancer. If you eat well, live healthy, and take necessary precautions, then you raise your chance of remaining cancer-free and never expressing that gene. The same holds true for anything else. I do believe that there is a genetic component to autism, but it won't necessarily express itself if you take precautions with food, environmental exposure, and chemicals. An aware parent can increase their child's likelihood of wellness without a diagnosis.

Building Blocks:

The Marsh family was a blended family. Mom and Dad entered into the marriage with two children each. The father's son, Patrick, was diagnosed with autism, and the mother's daughter, Rose, was also diagnosed on the spectrum. The mom brought Rose to see me after hearing about biomedical interventions, and I began a very successful treatment with her.

Then, the Marsh family grew with the addition of a beautiful baby girl. In knowing the family history on both sides, I expressed a concern for the new baby and began treating her at four months using the very principles being taught in this book. The baby is now two and is very healthy and developing wonderfully. She is definitely on the right path. The genetic statistics are not in her favor, but how the Marsh family raises her and supports her development just may make the difference. I only hope more families seek preventative care in the future so there is a decline in ASD diagnoses.

Since medical experts are focused on the fact that autism is due to genetics, they have limited the choices of medications and treatments to only those that manage the symptoms. Those who suffer from autism take psychotropic drugs or medications that affect one's central nervous system, altering brain functions, and they undergo therapy to correct a number of symptoms caused by the disorder, such as obsessive and anti-social behaviors. These medications do not cure autism; instead, they are more like maintenance procedures, akin to taking out the garbage. Well, why don't doctors and parents stop the trash from accumulating in the first place? These medications have side effects that can range from seizures, excessive weight gain, insomnia, stomach pain, and headaches. Unfortunately, many parents of non-verbal children have no idea that they are adding to the physical pains of their child. Some children with autism are good candidates for medication, but would actually do much better with proper biomedical care.

Seeking biomedical care will never make matters worse (if you seek a quality doctor), and know that medication will always be an option on the table—so perhaps it can wait. You may be able to improve your child's health and well-being without medication or at a minimal dose that regulates them. I always hope for the best: a drug-free child who can be happy, healthy, and enjoying life without pain.

Asperger's (AKA Aspy)

Asperger's syndrome is commonly known as the "high functioning" form of autism. As a result, many parents of aspy children are not as supported as those with lower functioning children on the autism spectrum. Parents of children on the severe end of the spectrum think a child with Asperger's is not as much work, but this is a false assumption. It is just as difficult, only with different challenges. Aspy children exhibit symptoms such as:

- Difficulties in social interaction
- Restricted and repetitive patterns of behavior and interests
- Physical clumsiness

- Atypical use of language
- Obsessive tendencies
- Lack of common sense
- Repetitive or scripted speech patterns
- Lack of attention
- Problems with organization

Although they do not have clinically significant delays in cognitive development or a general delay in language, children with Asperger's have intense behaviors. As a matter of fact, most exhibit high IQs and sophisticated vocabularies. These children display behavior, interests, and activities that are restricted, repetitive, and abnormally intense or focused. It is not uncommon to see an aspy child collect volumes of detailed information on a relatively narrow topic without having genuine understanding of the broader topic. For example, in history class kids learn the U.S. presidents, and an aspy may find this very interesting and begin to study them. In doing so, they will get very detailed in their knowledge of presidents' lives, but when asked about how that plays into history in the broader sense, they revert back to the specific details they may know while ignoring the bigger picture. They will fixate and only want to speak about what they like or enjoy. Needless to say it can be a challenge for the parents and educators.

Building Blocks:

Vickie was a freshman in high school when she came strolling into my life with her mom. She was confident in her knowledge, but very introverted in general unless you asked her about her interests. Knowing she had Asperger's, I explained that she was seeing me for nutrition and asked her if she knew anything about it. She shyly looked up and shook her head no. I then asked her if she could research the supplements I was giving her and let me know what she thought about them the following week. Vickie was excited and agreed. My plan was to get her on my side, gaining an interest in her own health to create more compliance. The following week she went into great detail, so much so that I could barely get a comment in. She seemed to talk for 30 minutes straight. Vickie was excited as we began our journey together, always educating each other on her care and addressing her concerns. This is a great way to build relationships with these kids and have them accept help. Children with Asperger's are very strong-willed and will not comply when they do not want to; I find they comply perfectly when you get them involved and empower them to help.

Aspys have difficulty with social interaction that is multidimensional. They do not understand social cues in general and find it hard to empathize, reciprocate emotion, and read nonverbal behaviors such as facial expressions. What all this adds up to is that they can be socially awkward. When talking, their speech can be somewhat incoherent and can include the echoing of a movie or show they often watch. Children with Asperger's don't look for interest from the other person when talking because they are too distracted with the facts and accuracy of what they are saying to realize that you are bored to death. This lack of engagement makes it hard for them to have relationships.

Building Blocks:

Kayla was diagnosed with Asperger's, and as she was growing up, it was harder and harder for her parents to help her. She was approaching her twelfth birthday, and her social awkwardness was at an all-time high. Kayla was guilty of blurting out what was on her mind; her mom told me that one time when they were shopping for groceries Kayla loudly asked, "Why is that lady fat?" Now, this is funny after the fact, but how do you explain to a perfect stranger that your child at twelve doesn't know better? Kayla, like most aspys, does not understand politeness, cannot read facial expressions, does not get jokes or humor, and doesn't have "common sense." This is a continual struggle, especially because she is an only child with no siblings to model after.

My suggestion to Kayla's mother was to seek out social skills training for her. Aspys do not know the basics of social cues, but because they are so very intelligent, they can be taught. These cues may come across as a bit robotic at times, but it's better for them to learn how to blend in with society as they get older since this is how they gain independence. It is also imperative for them to learn when someone may be taking advantage of them, as well as what is proper, especially physically, as they get older. The social skills training classes that combine aspys and "normal" children are most successful because children with Asperger's can model behavior they see in other kids their age, and it also forces them to socialize, which is often not a priority on their list. Kayla attended her classes, and I began to see a confidence in her that wasn't there before. Plus, her parents and I felt better knowing there was a safe place for her to experience the awkwardness and learn options on how to handle social interaction in the future.

Unlike children with autism who prefer to be alone, aspys may get involved and will say whatever is on their mind. Sometimes parents joke that they have no filter, like Kayla, and I would have to agree. Everything is very literal to them, so humor, irony, and teasing often go right over their heads. Instead they will laugh when everyone else laughs without having a true understanding of what the others find so funny. Many aspy children are very immature for their age when it comes to social communication. This can improve with age and lots of coaching, but some things will always persist, becoming part of their personalities. I often coach my parents to think like their child, to take everything literally and then break things down so they can see the logic. While incredibly intelligent, aspys have a different perspective and therefore grasp information in a unique way.

Building Blocks:

I previously introduced you to Vickie, and this story is perhaps one of the best examples I have to share. She was the baby of her family, and with so many siblings in the house, the mornings were a mad rush for Mom. Vickie attended private school and was required to wear a uniform daily. Every morning her mom would ask her to get dressed, brush her teeth, and so on. Mom was frustrated because, despite having the same routine for years, Vickie still could not get through a morning without her mother prodding her with directions. Vickie would get dressed some mornings and put on dirty clothes, or black socks when she was required to wear white socks, and had been doing so for fourteen years, an obvious annoyance to Mom.

I simply explained to her mom that, because Vickie had Asperger's, her mind works much differently. I suggested she write a list of "Morning To-Do's" and post it in Vickie's bedroom, bathroom, and kitchen since these are the places she visited each morning. An aspy will typically do amazing with a bit of direction via a list, or photos for those who do not read yet. You see their minds click with a list, and that keeps parents from having to repeat things over and over again. The medical community has established that they are brilliant, but they lack the processing to remember more than two to three items or commands at a time. This is why something as simple as getting ready for school is a nightmare. You can try making a list of steps for any routine and see the anxiety lessen as directions get followed. This empowers these children to be independent and successful.

When deciding on treatment, I find it best to look at the biomedical reasons for these symptoms. Just as in the case with autism, these children have other deficiencies and medical issues to address. I have seen countless children diagnosed with Asperger's syndrome who had longstanding behavioral problems, digestive issues, picky eating habits, abnormal bowels, and poor sleep. Doctors and society place more focus on autism being treatable than on Asperger's, but remember that they belong on the same spectrum and can therefore both be treated.

I have also seen social skills groups help these children greatly, as with Kayla. Social skills training courses are usually run by a therapist (OT, PhD, etc.). The goal is to teach "proper" social cues, conversation, and interaction in public, among many other everyday skills. The cognitive ability of children with Asperger's often allows them to articulate social cues in this context. They can gain a theoretical understanding of other people's emotions and apply this knowledge in real-life situations.

ADD/ADHD

Now let's focus on some of the most diagnosed delays, ADD and ADHD. Many children do not meet all the qualifications for an ADD or ADHD label. In some cases Asperger's, autism, sensory processing disorder, and learning disabilities are factors that may be overlooked. The diagnosis of ADD and ADHD is rampant among children, and they are often misdiagnosed.

These children are at the highest risk for prescription psychotropic drugs and depression. The mask of the drugs can sometimes be helpful for families until they begin to realize that the real issue involves the whole system. The answer is not in medicating symptoms, but healing the body by finding the source of the problem. There are few children that truly need medication for these disorders, but many more can be helped without the use of these dangerous medications.

In ADD, a problem with inattention affects daily tasks, and symptoms can include:

- Poor ability with details
- Difficulty sustaining attention
- Frequently fails to listen carefully
- Does not follow directions
- Poor organization
- Losing things often
- Hard time completing tasks
- Easily distracted
- Forgetful

ADHD is a bit different because it also involves hyperactivity and impulsiveness. These children have symptoms such as:

- Cannot remain seated at school
- Restless, disruptive
- Talking excessively
- Poor memory
- Sleep problems
- Oppositional defiance disorder
- Difficulty awaiting their turn
- Interrupting conversations
- Tantrums and outbursts
- Poor gross and fine motor skills, such as handwriting and coordination
- Difficult time with transitions and changes to routine

Some physicians consider children with ADD or ADHD to be on the autism spectrum because they share commonalities such as speech difficulties, anxiety, mood disorders, depression, learning disabilities, sleep issues, communication problems, and obsessive-compulsive tendencies.

The root of the problem is in nutritional deficiencies, the body's ability to detoxify, inflammation, hormone irregularities, and digestion. I see more children misdiagnosed with ADD and ADHD that actually have food allergies; the food is making their bodies short circuit. If your child has these symptoms or has been diagnosed with ADD or ADHD, it would be a good idea to look a bit deeper into what may be the root cause in order to repair the things that have gone off track. Many times ADD and ADHD are easy to treat and require a smaller commitment as compared to other developmental delays.

Processing Disorders

I would be remiss if I didn't touch on processing disorders as these are often interlaced with the other spectrum disorders. The most commonly talked about processing disorder is sensory processing disorder, or SPD; this also encompasses the prior name sensory integration disorder/dysfunction. Sensory processing is an important job for the nervous system, and the signals need to transmit and organize information in order for a person to process and use it correctly. Sometimes there is heavy traffic in the transmission, and messages don't get correctly organized. This is the premise of a processing disorder. There are five senses to consider: touch, sight, taste, smell, and hearing. This disorder is vast in its manifestations, so it is frequently misdiagnosed or not diagnosed at all.

Many children have sound or auditory sensitivities. These are the kids that may wear headphones to keep noise at a minimum. Parents often struggle to go to busy and loud places with these children because it is auditory overload for them. The auditory threshold is impaired in these kids, and they will often stretch out words while talking, echo, or repeat themselves. When hearing sounds, it is much like a bad cell phone connection to them. Children with auditory problems exhibit dyslexia, oppositional defiance, and autism spectrum disorders.

Visual processing can also be affected as part of SPD, and these kids will tilt their head, avoid escalators and fluorescent lighting, examine fingers closely, and have trouble catching a ball. When reading, the words can jiggle or vibrate, which breaks up the visual images, making it hard to consistently see how words should appear. But, these children's eye exams will be normal. Sight itself isn't the problem; the information the brain receives from the eyes is scrambled. There are ways to help visually affected SPD children at home: block or remove fluorescent lights, use a laptop computer, favor a desk lamp over the overhead light, and print on pastel paper. Consult with your occupational therapist for home exercises for your child's specific needs.

Building Blocks

Sometimes SPD can manifest in odd ways, at least to most people looking in from the outside. A seven-year-old boy's parents brought him into my office and described his terrible fear of hand dryers, those super loud blowing machines found on the wall in public bathrooms. Most families that have this experience, especially with such a distinct fear, just think their child is weird and do not know to ask for a medical opinion. In many cases those noises are painful to SPD children, and they are not just throwing a tantrum—they are in pain. I educated the boy's parents on SPD and asked them to get an evaluation from their school to make sure this was not an issue. Sure enough, he was diagnosed and was able to get the therapy he needed.

In treating kids with SPD, it is really important to take a multidisciplinary approach, addressing biomedical issues as well as treating the physical issues with craniosacral therapy. I have found CST to be one of the most beneficial therapies for kids with SPD because it balances out the two parts of the nervous system (sympathetic and parasympathetic), aiding it in calming down and transmitting information correctly. By removing the system irritation, you can allow their senses to stay out of overdrive.

The most prevalent form of SPD, tactile or touch defensiveness can be hardest for parents. These children are often fearful and anxious when being touched, even as infants. Many parents never physically bond with a child that has tactile SPD. These kids will complain about brushing their hair, rough sheets or clothes, and certain textures. Water or messy play activities may be torture for them, and they can be distressed by dirt and certain foods. This tactile response can be hyporesponsive (weaker) or hyperresponsive (stronger). Some hyporesponsive kids will love to be hugged super tight and may even pinch or scratch themselves to feel sensory input. Many parents see huge changes when desensitizing their child. This is an important thing to do for kids so that they can enjoy affection and develop feelings of kindness. An occupational therapist can use brushing, swinging, weighted vest, or pressure therapy to calm the nervous system down, and they can teach things you can do at home to help.

I have found medically that these children are also fragile and suffer with GI issues, food sensitivities, and deficiencies. When these issues are left untreated, a child will many times stop progressing in therapy, hitting a plateau instead of recovering fully. I have found the most successful treatment to be a combination of biomedical interventions with craniosacral and occupational therapies.

Building Blocks:

Adrian and David are brothers who both had SPD, but their manifestations were very different. Both boys are very outgoing, playful, and intelligent. By the time I met the family, their mom had been through the ringer trying to get help. This was hard because she was so educated on her children's condition. After seeing the boys get worse with biomedical treatment, she was obviously hesitant to continue, so she decided to take another route and came to me for CST.

Adrian did not like to be touched, would take hours to get dressed in the morning because he could not stand clothing, was sensitive to odors, hated haircuts, and had food texture issues. These problems also made Adrian very moody, and he would back off in social situations even when he wanted to engage just because he was overwhelmed. David, on the other hand, suffered with tremendous anxiety, had extreme OCD about hand washing, and had very limiting food texture issues.

I began CST on both boys, and the results were amazing to see. To watch them blossom was great for us all. After a few weeks of treatment, Dad came in and told me Adrian had asked him to rub his back, which he would never have done in the past. He also did not mind haircuts and was dealing much better with clothing, noise, and anxiety. David was calmer and easier to soothe. After their CST treatments were complete, none of the sensory issues were concerns, and both were doing wonderfully.

Of course, the biomedical end of this situation needed to be dealt with sooner or later to address their food issues and other complaints, so Mom entrusted me to begin working on them biomedically. And things just kept getting better. David previously suffered from terrible eczema, which caused him great pain, and to feel this improving made him so happy. These boys were some of the sweetest patients, and shortly after beginning their treatment, David came to me to say, "Thank you, Dr. Brooks," and gave me a huge hug. Those are the moments I live for. They make me so proud of the parents I work with and their commitment to helping heal their children.

The list of symptoms and categories is massive when delving into sensory processing disorder. I always refer my families to an occupational therapist who has experience in sensory integration and uses a sensory gym in treatment. When I am caring for the underlying medical issues and the occupational therapist handles the physical ones, the team as a whole is able to make huge strides in recovery for these SPD children.

Chapter 9: ABCs of Lab Testing

It is important that parents understand that lab testing is there to provide information; this does not mean every doctor out there has all the knowledge needed to order the necessary tests for this precious population. In fact, many parents come to me after years of testing and having doctors tell them there is nothing wrong or that nothing can be done to help. It is imperative to find a biomedical, functional, or integrative care physician to work with to increase the likelihood of getting the proper tests and in turn achieving recovery for your child.

There are many lab options to choose from, and your pediatrician or GI doctor may only order tests that are covered under your insurance. However, the specialty tests that need to be done are often out-of-network. Parents often inquire if labs can be ordered locally to have them covered or assume that if their pediatrician orders them they are covered, but this is false. It doesn't matter what doctor orders the labs or where the lab is located if the lab company itself is not in your insurance company's network. This insurance game is a nightmare for us all; the labs do not get enough money reimbursed by your insurance companies to cover the cost of the test, so they cannot afford to accept the amount allowed by an insurance company. Parents should know that doctors who regularly treat children with delays or special needs do not run tests that cannot be used to help with recovery. I myself don't ask a family to pay for labs I cannot use or will not use to help them in the very best way.

Many doctors, including myself, do provide take-home stool and urine testing for parents as well as preliminary blood work. The blood work may be abundant the first time as doctors like to get answers about what is currently happening as well as baseline numbers for future sickness or deficiency. There are places where parents can order tests without a doctor, but I recommend not doing this unless you have someone to interpret the labs for you. The labs results are meaningless if interpreted incorrectly. Reading these lab reports is complicated, and any great doctor doesn't just look at what is out of normal limits. Biomedical doctors piece together a clinical picture using all of the available data and present the results to you clearly. Most pediatricians do not know of these specialty labs; they just weren't in their toolbox in medical school, nor is this the current standard of care.

Building Blocks:

I do not have specific instance to point out involving lab work because this is an issue with everyone. Some people come to me with years of previous tests; some are useful, and some are not. The biggest concern to me is the lack of proper care and/or improper following of the treatment plan. It is easy for me to blame another doctor if I see things that should have been dealt with, but many times it's the parents who cancel appointments, do not follow directions, and in turn fall off the wagon.

Some parents do this because they do not understand the test results and therefore do not see the necessity for change, while others get improvement and become complacent and never follow through until another issue arises that must be dealt with by their doctor. My advice is to always find someone you feel comfortable with, trust, and can be open with. Every treatment has tough moments, and you need to be able to communicate both the good and bad. When a family actively works with their doctor, the results can be life-changing.

Interpretation is VITAL in Recovery

I want to touch on interpretation and the role it plays in your child's recovery. When I refer to "interpretation," I am speaking to the act of the physician looking over your medical history, ordering proper labs, and recommending appropriate treatments based on your individual child. This is vital in any care plan and for every single child. It is also important to understand that a biomedical or functional medicine doctor takes much more time to review your results and prepare this interpretation because he or she has a primary goal of solving the core issues, which requires putting all the pieces together, no matter how slow the process. There are times I have thirty-plus pages to go through, and I rework my entire treatment plan based on those results; this cannot be done in two minutes, nor should it be. Most doctors all but glance at your lab results before entering the room and are reviewing them with you for that brief two minutes before shoveling you out the door; this is the most common model in our medical system. Common or not, which type of doctor do you want treating your child?

I have had hundreds of patients say, "Dr. Brooks, my other doctor never ran that test," or, "My doctor didn't tell me what the labs meant." Now, just because your doctor doesn't review labs with you doesn't mean they were not interpreted—BUT you as the parent need to understand the results in terms that are simple. What is happening with your child, and what is going to be done (especially at home) to fix things?

Look at it this way: When you take your car in for repairs, they give it a look, write a quote, and repair the car. When you pick it up, they detail what was done and explain things to you in basic terms, so you leave understanding why your car was making that clunking noise and perhaps ways to avoid it in the future. Now, let's say you brought your car in for repairs and they didn't give you a quote or take a look, but just asked for the keys. Then you went to pick up the car, and they just asked for your payment without another word. Would you understand why you just paid them a bunch of money? No, you would leave not knowing what was wrong with your car or ways to avoid future damage. In fact, many of you would never return. Am I right?

Unfortunately, doctor appointments work this way too. People keep going back to doctors who don't spend the time they need with patients to help them understand. What happens when you do that as a parent? Your child's recovery is slower or absent. Most parents will not comply because it takes a lot of work to get their child better, and when they don't fully grasp the why behind the rules, it's hard to follow them. Not to mention parents are left feeling unsure of whether or not they really need the rules.

Parents who get the best results do two things: (1) they are consistent with the treatment plan, which includes follow-up appointments with the doctor, and (2) they understand the problems facing their child and are dedicated to the treatment plan. It sounds simple, and it can be, depending on your journey and who you choose to be on your team.

So let's get back to interpretation. As you probably know by now, everyone has an opinion, and interpretation is no different. However, experience and specialty matter when it comes to these children, who I consider to be medically fragile. Each doctor will interpret things differently, and this is where choice comes in for parents. The key ingredient in gaining recovery is examining the child as a whole, not zeroing in on one part that is not functioning. When your child has an ear infection, the general practitioner or specialist just looks at the ears. When the infections become chronic, only then do they begin to think perhaps there is a larger issue. Instead, doctors should dig down to the root of the problem when the first infection occurs and keep that child from getting recurring infections to begin with—that is the huge difference between traditional and functional medicine.

My job (as well as any physician's) is to look at the whole child, not just the portion that appears to not be working right. Let's go back to the car example. If you take your car to the mechanic for a clanking sound in your engine, do they just look under the hood, or do they look at any and all components that could create the noise you described? Any quality mechanic would look at the car as a whole and rule out potential sources of the noise. The body should be looked at as a whole, too, because where the clanking noise in the body originates is not always as obvious as it seems. The body is a whole, all parts affecting one another, so why ignore any of it?

Once a doctor realizes that a child's symptoms are a small part of a larger issue, the next step is ordering proper lab testing. Many of the labs that functional medicine/biomedical doctors order are specialty tests designed to look for very specific things, hence why your general practitioner never uses them. Lastly, the doctor interprets the labs in part based on the history received from the family, so please be honest when reporting medical data.

The lab companies try to help physicians by giving an interpretation, but this is often vague and not specific to age or diagnosis. They also flag high and low scores that occur outside of the normal range, BUT decoding the data from a lab is not that simple. For example, a high or low normal value (not flagged) can still be abnormal and can have a direct correlation to a symptom your child is experiencing. It's a bad habit doctors have when reviewing labs; they just look at the abnormal column on labs and don't really look at the clinical picture or at the borderline high or low values. Things can easily be avoided symptomatically if caught early, so why not look at everything, big and small?

Building Blocks:

When labs are ordered, make sure to ask if you will have an opportunity to sit down and review them in laymen's terms with the doctor so you can really grasp what is happening. Please be prepared to pay for this extra time as many doctors book appointments every fifteen minutes, which is most likely not enough time for a thorough review. I assure you the money you spend to sit with your doctor will be well worth it. Bring a pad of paper and pen to the appointment because many doctors, including myself, do not allow tape recordings of appointments to ensure patient privacy. If your doctor recommends a referral based on the results, ask that they provide you with a letter to that specialist explaining the need for additional testing or treatment. Why? Not every doctor can read and understand these tests, so you want to ensure your doctors are on the same page. This will help them communicate with one another and work together to provide the best care possible.

At the end of the day, recovery is all about putting a puzzle together. All the pieces of a child's life, their experiences and medical concerns, have to be considered to see the big picture. You must have a doctor who gives your child the necessary attention beginning at the first visit, ordering proper labs, and most important, offering the experience and expertise to evaluate the lab results and make proper recommendations. If you miss something, even minor, it can make a world of difference for a child. You know your child is more sensitive and aware; this is a huge part of it. Their bodies are more reactive, and therefore the smallest things missed during interpretation can hinder them from really achieving recovery.

It's like the old saying: beauty is in the eye of the beholder. The labs, interpretation, and complete history make for a successful treatment plan. For me, "recovery is in the hands of the beholder," and it ultimately depends on your goals and the doctor you choose to take the journey with you. If your physician has the knowledge to read, interpret, and really look at your whole child as one entity, then you have a great shot at getting fantastic results.

Of course, finding a great doctor is only half the battle because you as the parent have to follow the treatment plan. Many times the doctor can answer the questions about what's happening and why, if pieced together completely, but they need your compliance to make this happen.

Chapter 10: Recovery

In a blink of an eye, your entire life changes with your child's diagnosis. This overwhelms every family, and most have little guidance. The maze of the Internet becomes the constant as parents search online for hope. Some parents get the care they need, whereas others spend ten years following dead ends. It is my mission to see parents get ALL their options for treatment. I cannot count the number of parents I've seen cry in frustration and in joy—frustration because no one told them about biomedical interventions, nutrition, or supplementation, and joy because they found the right team and are relieved to be getting their child on the right track. Parents do not have to go without guidance or options, but when they do, recovery is bleak.

The team you select to help your child may be one of the most important decisions of your child's recovery, and who you choose to treat your child is no small matter. I often joke with my patients' mothers and tell them they have the right to interview and ask questions of anyone who is a potential team member, just like they interviewed every man they dated until they found their mate. Just like finding your spouse or partner, this will affect your daily life going forward. The attributes to look for include someone who spends the necessary time to learn about your child and explain to you as the parents what is happening. By working together, a treatment strategy can evolve.

Most of the medical profession treats symptoms with therapy or drugs. As a result, the underlying issue goes unresolved, and the child remains unwell. Families need compassion, understanding, and experience from their providers, and if you do your research and interview candidates for your child's medical team based on your goals and needs, you will find the right doctors and therapists to help your family.

I hear about "recovery" for autism and other delays, is this possible?

ABSOLUTELY. I can say that not only from my own experience, but also from the medical data that backs up these interventions. I always say that recovery depends on the child and goals. Each child is different, and therefore every individual's recovery looks different. Through the years, I have seen a positive correlation between those who are consistent with medical care, dietary changes, supplements, and therapy. The body needs consistency; it's very hard to pinpoint the "breaking point" for each individual. Have you ever noticed poor behavior or your child not feeling well after eating a certain food? That's the breaking point that cannot always be measured. The body's reaction to an insult is just as important as a fancy test. My advice to parents is always to be consistent to yield the best recovery possible. Some children are more sensitive than others, as many parents can attest, so consistency is very important. The testing doctors have available today helps guide treatment, but parental feedback is equally important. Like I said before, recovery is all about putting a puzzle together, so I created a puzzle model that you can follow to piece together your child's recovery.

Recovery Model

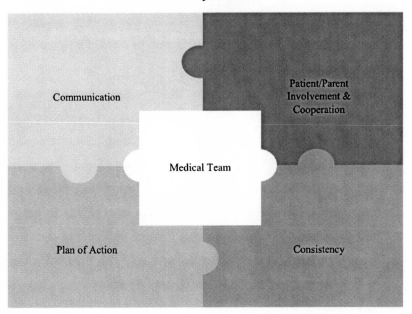

Key:

- **Medical Team:** This is the team of experts you have chosen to help guide you. It may include your biomedical doctor, therapists (occupational/speech), counselor, and school administrators/ teachers.

- **Communication:** This is key, and all parties involved with your child should be willing to provide communication in a team approach to ensure the best result. If you come across someone who is not a team player, please give a second thought to working with him or her as it could deter your child from reaching recovery.

- **Patient/Parent Involvement and Cooperation:** This responsibility mostly falls on the parents. It's important to make sure that each parent or guardian is on the same page following the consistency needed in the treatment plan to achieve success. Part of this is making sure to see your doctor regularly for scheduled follow-ups. The doctor cannot help you if you do not go in to discuss things, nor can they update the treatment plan as needed to keep your child on track.

- **Consistency:** This is perhaps the biggest component in failed treatment because the parents get off track and then spiral out of care, cutting off any progress achieved and stunting future improvement.

- **Plan of Action:** Start this by making a list of goals for treatment, and then devise a plan with each member of your team and with your family. I find this action plan helps keep things in perspective and gives you that much-needed light at the end of the tunnel to focus on when you are getting burned out. This plan will change, so be flexible and understand that change does not always have to be a bad thing.

Take time right now to write down five goals you have for your child, and get to work on envisioning those coming to fruition. The next step is to find a physician to help guide you on your journey. Remember: it's much easier with help! The most successful parents are the ones who reach out for help and support. The others get discouraged and lose steam, and that never heals a child.

Chapter 11: Treatment Options

Treatment options vary widely depending on your child's diagnosis or symptoms and who you choose for your treatment team. Traditionally, when a family is told that their child has a developmental delay, the next step is a referral to a speech and/or occupational therapist. These two therapies are the most mainstream and widely understood. Speech therapy can be a critical part of aiding your child with articulation, fluency, resonance, dysphasia, and receptive and expressive language. Occupational therapy helps children with motor skills for self-care, work, and daily living. Some occupational therapists have additional education in sensory disorders and can be a huge help with these challenges.

The next several sections will outline other therapies worth knowing about and will list several others that are not discussed in depth. I urge you to do your research and have a good understanding of your child's needs and which professionals may be the best fit to help.

Biomedical Care

There are inaccuracies among parents about the definition and uses of biomedical intervention. The biomedical approach is based on the latest scientific research showing biological causes, such as heavy metal poisoning, yeast infection, food sensitivity, gastrointestinal dysfunction, and nutritional deficiency. This new understanding has brought new hope to children and their families. Parents are often told that their child's diagnosis is the result of genetics and is psychological in nature. Typical psychological manifestations in children may include delayed speech, lack of eye contact, impaired or non-present social skills, shyness, stimming, delayed gross or fine motor skills, sensory integration issues (e.g., sound and touch sensitivity), not responding to one's name, inflexibility with transitions, and major, often unexplained, changes in mood.

The physical or medical issues children often manifest are rarely noted or discussed. Your doctor should examine the typical physical manifestations including food allergies, eczema, general gastrointestinal distress, constipation and diarrhea, yeast overgrowth, immune system dysregulation, and sleep disturbances to help in the treatment of the whole child. Biomedical intervention is based on the belief that the psychological symptoms are a product of the physical issues the child is experiencing and that addressing the physical issues will lead to an improvement in those psychological symptoms.

Most people have heard of biomedical care for children with autism, but in my experience, it's clear that any child with developmental delays should be treated using biomedical care. It addresses the core of the problem, and that is what is needed in treatment regardless of diagnosis. Remember that getting to the core of the issues is one of the keys in recovery and is part of your medical team's responsibility. Parents play an active role as well and must dig deep and have faith when they are getting to the root cause of what ails their child.

Building Blocks:

When a child is having issues, most parents look to traditional means of care, and for some families, this resolves the problem. The larger majority suffer for years unaware of their options. I have seen children initially improve in traditional therapy and then start to plateau. Parents who decide to do biomedical care reap huge rewards, seeing the plateau disappear and new goals start to be achieved. I have too many stories to tell in this regard. Parents come in with children who are in therapy 40 hours a week and still not seeing recovery. Then they introduce biomedical care, and POOF!— their child comes alive and gets back on the road to recovery. In the end, it helps the therapist, the family, and most importantly the child.

Nutrition

Parents often assume that their child is properly nourished. Pediatric nutrition does not follow a one-size-fits-all philosophy. Just as each child is unique, so is the proper nutritional balance for each child. Through the use of laboratory tests, your doctor should be able to create highly individualized nutritional and supplemental advisement.

Caregivers and parents must teach children nutritional intelligence from an early age. For example, give your children options for food, but ensure that all choices are healthy, wholesome, and organic. This enables children to participate by allowing choices that will empower them. As they grow older, they will continue making healthy choices, even when you are not around to control the options. The foods in their diet should be healing in nature, and it is important to introduce this concept to your child at an early age. The appreciation for healthy foods may keep your child from suffering from digestive challenges such as constipation/diarrhea, deficiencies in vitamins and minerals, and failure to thrive, as well as ensuring they don't become picky eaters.

Some parents are faced with the challenges of raising a special needs child. Special needs children are often nutritionally imbalanced, craving foods that feed dysfunction in the gut. This leads to poor behaviors, stimming, inadequate sleep, and severe digestive challenges, to name a few symptoms. My advice is that you address the nutritional components of illness and initiate the healing process through the use of proper nutrition.

A parent must have an abundant amount of information to address nutritional deficiencies. I know firsthand the challenges of making these changes and spend the necessary time to educate each parent with the tools to make this transition as smooth as possible. It is important to get guidance with your child's nutrition at every step to ensure proper growth and development. There are many facets of a child's nutrition to be discussed with your doctor or nutritionist, but the following are a few aspects that I feel most strongly about:

Food Sensitivity/Specific Diets: Many children have problems with digestion, including food sensitivity—particularly to casein in dairy and gluten in wheat products. Your doctor will prescribe dietary changes targeted specifically for the needs of your child.

Yeast/Bacterial Overgrowth: Children commonly suffer from yeast (Candida) and other bacterial overgrowth in their intestines. This could arise from several sources, the most common being the excessive use of antibiotics. Yeast interferes with the absorption of food, leading to failure to thrive, poor behavior, picky eating, and severe cravings. Proper testing needs to be done to identify the problems prior to treatment.

Minerals and Vitamins: A large majority of children are deficient in minerals and vitamins such as zinc, magnesium, iodine, potassium, vitamin C, and B vitamins. It is important to eat foods rich in these nutrients, particularly organic foods, as much as possible. These deficiencies can be addressed with high potency vitamin/mineral supplements to achieve the adequate balance necessary for your child.

Building Blocks:

I have yet to find no nutritional issues after running labs on a child. Perhaps this is due to our over-processed food sources, or the fact that parents are always on the go and cook less than previous generations. Either way, every child needs to be evaluated to make sure nutrition is being optimized. Why not ensure that your children are maximizing their health?

Chiropractic

Ever have your family doctor or pediatrician enter the room for two minutes and never make eye contact? I've heard this complaint from mothers for years. This is how chiropractors like myself are different. Chiropractors invest in someone's wellness. This includes talking about hobbies, relationships, and work. Chiropractors know how these things affect your health, and this also gives us an opportunity to get to know you individually. I can't tell you how many times I've been asked, "Dr. Brooks, why didn't my doctor tell me that?" In short, it's because they didn't take the time to talk, to educate, and mostly to listen. I couldn't function without knowing my patients. My success would be minimal and my practice a failure.

As a Board Certified Pediatric Chiropractor, I have a love for chiropractic and all its healing power. Chiropractors have been caring for children for more than 100 years, and chiropractic treatment has proven to benefit children with chronic infections, pain, and delays. Many of the common childhood ailments will also respond to this safe, natural form of health care. Parents, especially those already receiving chiropractic care themselves, are seeking out the same safe care for their children. Each of the children I see gets to benefit from chiropractic care, and they love it.

The word chiropractic comes from the Greek word *chiropraktikos*, meaning "treatment by hand." This is exactly what chiropractors do: use their hands to adjust the body to promote healing and wellness. Modern chiropractic treatment began in 1895 when Daniel David Palmer delivered the first recorded chiropractic adjustment to Harvey Lillard, a janitor in his office. Harvey had been deaf since suffering a back injury during childhood. Harvey had a full recovery from his back pain, including the restoration of his hearing, after only that one adjustment. Although this is an extreme example, and chiropractic is certainly not a usual cure for deafness, Dr. Palmer's story clearly illustrates the potential that chiropractic care demonstrates within the realm of healing.

On the surface it may seem that chiropractic is limited, but that's not always the case. The spine's function is to provide protection to the spinal cord, which is a direct extension of the brain. The brain and spinal cord are complex and delicate, yet responsible for running and maintaining all the systems and functions of the body. You can think of the spinal cord as the wires that enable the brain to communicate with all parts of the body. Like the brain is encased in the skull, the spinal cord is encased in the vertebrae. The vertebrae afford protection to the delicate spinal cord while allowing for a full range of motion.

The spine is made up of several joints, and each one of these joints must be moving entirely and properly in all of its ranges of motion. If even one of the joints is not moving properly, it disturbs the balance and alignment of the body. The lack of proper movement of these vertebral joints is called spinal fixation (subluxation). When a vertebral joint is not moving properly, this imbalance disturbs the nervous system. A chiropractor is trained to correct subluxations or fixations of the spine through a process known as chiropractic adjustment. The adjustments on children are very gentle, often using just the fingertips, and kids enjoy learning about their bodies throughout the process.

The chiropractic philosophy is based on the following belief statements:

1. All bodily functions are connected, and the healing process involves the entire body.

2. A healthy nervous system, particularly the spine, is the key to a healthy body.

   The spinal cord carries information throughout the body and is responsible for all bodily functions. When the systems of the body are in balance, it is called *homeostasis*. Disorders of the bones, muscles, and nerves can disrupt homeostasis and increase the risk of disease and other health problems.

3. When body systems are in harmony, the human body has the remarkable ability to maintain health and heal itself.

Common childhood disorders can also be linked with spinal dysfunction, these include:

- Acid reflux (GERD)
- ADD/ADHD
- Allergies/sinus problems
- Asthma
- Bedwetting and/or constipation
- Colic

- Digestive problems
- Growing pains
- Headaches
- Persistent sore throat, coughs, or colds
- Recurrent ear infections
- Scoliosis
- Torticollis
- And many more....

Some chiropractors are taught about pediatrics in school, but usually only get a very broad overview. It is best to seek out care from a doctor who has additional training in pediatrics via post-graduate work. You can go to www.icpa4kids.com to look for a doctor in your area, BUT you will want to look for the proper initials after their name. The designations specific to a trained pediatric provider have changed through the years, but you will want to look for CACCP, DACCP, or FICPA; these mean the chiropractor has completed a two-year postgraduate training in pediatrics and pregnancy and has passed their boards in these areas. Other doctors are listed who are "members" and may be working on the designation but are not yet board certified. There are many qualified doctors to see, and in the end, the choice is up to you. This book has detailed much of the extended value that these pediatric specialists can bring to your child, and you'll likely find that their expertise is worth seeking out.

Building Blocks:

I try to educate parents about chiropractic care and the benefits that regular care can have to overall bodily function. Many children get ill with the occasional cold, fever, or ear infection, and this is just one time when an adjustment can truly work miracles. One of the many benefits to an adjustment is increasing lymphatic drainage, allowing toxins to flush out of the system. This becomes imperative with a cold, fever, or ear infection because all the fluids get stuck in the head and cannot drain out. In many cases a child can come in for an adjustment, and the fever will immediately break, followed by drainage and a quicker recovery from the cold or ear infection. Many chiropractors like myself will also give parents natural home care options to treat these common illnesses and help avoid the dreaded antibiotics.

Craniosacral Therapy

Craniosacral therapy (CST) was pioneered and developed by osteopathic physician John Upledger following extensive scientific studies from 1975 to 1983 at Michigan State University, where he served as a clinical researcher and professor of biomechanics. CST is a gentle, hands-on method of evaluating and enhancing the functioning of a physiological body system called the craniosacral system—comprised of the cranial bones, cerebrospinal fluid (CSF), and the membranes. The system works together to pump CSF throughout the system. The membranes surround the brain and spinal cord like a wetsuit, and the cranial bones sit on top.

These membranes can become restricted or wrinkled. When the tissue is wrinkled, the nerves that go through it get irritated, and symptoms result. Imagine your bed sheets upon waking in the morning; they are wrinkled from sleeping all night, and most of us wake up and fix the sheets to straighten them back out. This is the same premise with CST. The goal is to un-wrinkle the tissue (membrane), relaxing the nervous system and allowing for proper CSF flow.

CST is a very calm and relaxing therapy. Children can read, listen to music, watch TV, or play with their toys during a session. The practitioner will feel for the CST rhythm by placing their hands on the cranial bones using a soft touch, generally no greater than five grams, or about the weight of a nickel. Restrictions are released in the craniosacral system to improve the functioning of the central nervous system. The CST rhythm is the flow of cerebrospinal fluid (CSF) pumping from the head down through the spine. The CSF is produced within the brain itself and contracts at a normal rate of 6 to 12 cycles per minute, creating the rhythm.

The proper pumping of the CSF is important for our body. Its functions include:

- Removing waste and toxins from cerebral metabolism
- Protecting the brain and spinal cord
- Supplying nutrients to the nervous system

A person properly trained in the technique with a background in treating children should perform CST; there is a very high level of finesse required when working on children. The treatment is aimed at the membranes with the goal of helping improve flow and exchange of fluids. CST is not necessarily about realigning the cranial bones, although in cases such as plagiocephaly (misshapen cranial bones commonly referred to as "flat spots"), this treatment can help tremendously.

How does this therapy help children?
- Removes waste and toxins from cerebral metabolism (Many children today are having trouble detoxifying, and this aids in that process.)
- Supplies nutrients to the nervous system
- Releases tension in the body
- Balances the autonomic nervous system (ANS)

The nervous system imbalance is the key to why this helps so many children. The autonomic nervous system (ANS) has two branches: the sympathetic (fight or flight) and the parasympathetic (rest and digest), both of which affect our bodies greatly. Most parents will describe their child's behavior as "ramped up" or that "they cannot seem to relax," and this imbalance is why. The sympathetic nervous system is in overdrive, and CST helps balance it back out, thereby decreasing that overdrive feeling.

Symptoms of ANS dysfunction may include:
- Abnormal sweating
- Anxiety
- Bed-wetting
- Constipation and/or diarrhea
- Dark/light intolerance
- Detoxification issues
- Difficulty potty training
- Emotional instability
- Feeding problems
- Hyperactivity
- Inattention
- Nausea
- Poor social skills
- Sensory processing problems
- Sleep problems
- Tics
- Vomiting

I am often asked how CST can help with emotions or physical trauma. During a physical trauma, such as birth, the cranial bones can become "stuck" or restricted, creating tension on the brain and related nerves. When this tension is present, it can keep the body from functioning appropriately, leading to symptoms such as colic, constipation, acid reflux, nursing issues, sleeping difficulties, ear infections, and much more.

CST can be especially helpful for patients who have had to deal with trauma, both emotional and physical, at some point in their lives. The body can retain the emotional imprint from the trauma, leading to residual effects. These effects sometimes present themselves as physical ailments. CST can help children rid their bodies of these patterns using somatoemotional release (SER) techniques. This therapeutic process uses and expands on the principles of CST to help rid the mind and body of the residual effects of trauma. SER offers applications designed to enhance results using CST and other complementary therapies. Through SER, the patient does not need to analyze the problem to release it, and the patient can therefore be treated with more privacy than found in psychological therapies.

Building Blocks:

I often see newborn babies, and when a mother reports a breech (abnormal positioning of the baby in utero) or difficult labor, I always look for signs of trauma. One of the most common signs is decreased range of motion in the neck. During the labor process, an infant's neck may become stuck, and after birth it's uncomfortable for them to move fully. Parents often note that the child prefers a rotation to one side over the other. Shortly after the restricted movement, parents begin to notice the flat spot on their head. This flat spot is due to positioning and can be helped with CST. CST removes the restrictions, releasing the neck tension and allowing for proper movement of the neck. It also helps get the cranial bones back to proper function, so the flat spot begins to disappear. It is important to note that the range of motion will come back within a few weeks, but improvement to the flat spot may take longer; this is normal.

CST is an amazing therapy regardless of age and helps many children. I see a range of ages from newborns all the way through college students, and results are plentiful. In the past ten years, many more parents have taken notice of how CST can help with autism. According to Dr. Upledger, autism is related in part to a loss of flexibility and probable inflammation of the membrane layers surrounding the brain. Johns Hopkins studies show that there are increased levels of pro-inflammatory cytokines, neuroglial activation, and inflammatory changes in the CSF of children with autism. This basically means that children with autism have more inflammation than their non-autistic counterparts, resulting in restrictive forces on the brain tissue that can cause strain to the different brain structures. Dysfunction follows, but when the restrictions are removed, the brain tissue can flush out toxins and inflammation. This detoxification naturally elevates biochemical processing, increasing the functioning of neurological pathways. The idea is to increase detoxification and allow for proper processing in a child's body, encouraging better outcomes all around.

There is not one way for a child to get a CST restriction. This restriction can go all the way back to their birth, so depending on your child's history, you may uncover many reasons for the restrictions. Some of the most common reasons are:

- Breech birth
- Cesarean section
- Childhood falls
- Difficult labor
- Forceps delivery
- Infections/illness
- Multiple birth (twins, triplets)
- Self-injurious behaviors
- Stress to nervous system
- Surgery
- Trauma
- Vacuum extraction

Like speech or occupational therapy, there are varying degrees of how long CST treatment takes. Typically, the duration varies depending on age, previous trauma, and developmental needs. I usually see children for 30-minute appointments twice weekly for a period of time, then once weekly until the restrictions have been removed. Average care is about twelve weeks if done consistently. After the initial care, I see them once monthly and/or when they are sick to help with drainage, to adjust for growth spurts, and to keep things moving correctly. I always tell parents this is a short-term therapy with a long-term result.

By complementing the body's natural healing processes, CST is increasingly used as a preventive health measure for its ability to bolster resistance to disease, and it is effective for a wide range of medical problems associated with pain and dysfunction, including but not limited to:

- Acid reflux
- ADD/ADHD
- Allergies
- Anxiety
- Autism
- Chronic fatigue
- Chronic neck and back pain
- Colic
- Constipation
- Developmental delays
- Digestive problems
- Down syndrome ear infections
- Emotional difficulties
- Failure to thrive
- Head-banging
- Migraine headaches
- Physical/emotional abuse
- Plagiocephaly & brachycephaly
- Pregnancy
- Scoliosis
- Seizures
- Sensory processing problems

- Stress & tension-related problems
- Temporomandibular joint syndrome (TMJ)
- Torticollis
- Traumatic brain & spinal cord injuries

Equine Therapy (ET)

This is an interactive therapy that some children, especially those with social issues, benefit from. ET is an opportunity for a child to bond with horses and many times learn how to interact with other people. The medical field has long seen improvements in children with chronic conditions when they work with animals, and this therapy is an extension of that school of thought. Many major cities offer ET or are on waiting lists, so if this is something you are considering, then make an appointment to tour the nearest facility.

Social skills groups

This is a topic I feel very strongly about. As delayed children get older, they remove themselves socially, often because they are aware of their differences, creating much anxiety and social isolation. Local psychologists and facilities offering therapy will host social skills camps. It's important for the child to have a relationship with the person holding the class because trust is a huge factor in letting down their guard and actively participating. Unlike a neurotypical ("normal") kid, a child with delays may not pick up on social cues from others and therefore never learns how to behave or interact according to social norms. The best remedy for this is a social skills group in a safe, non-judgmental environment. My favorite groups will actually take the kids on outings during the meeting time, giving them "real life" experiences and, in turn, great social opportunities.

Hyperbaric Oxygen Therapy (HBOT)

This therapy uses 100% oxygen and requires the use of a pressure chamber. This is medically supervised, and an assessment is needed prior to delivery of HBOT. There are varying types of chambers, from hard to soft and even portable chambers that can be rented for use in the home. I feel strongly that a person should be medically supervised in a hard chamber when beginning this therapy. HBOT is primarily used for postsurgical, stroke and injury patients due to its inflammatory reducing properties. Now parents are also seeking out HBOT to reduce inflammation in their developmentally delayed child. There are varying degrees of efficacy with HBOT, according to which scientist you ask, but I have found it to help some patients by decreasing inflammation usually present throughout their body.

There are many therapies from neurological to interactive, and this is not my expertise, so I urge you to research these modalities and keep your physician informed of your findings. I simply covered the more common therapies, or those I use in practice myself. Be wary of any therapy center you choose for your child, and make sure that they will work well with your medical team. If they require you to drop out of every other treatment to partake of their therapy, take caution as this can be very damaging to a child, and in the end, no single therapy usually works. As they say, it takes a village to raise a child, and that includes supporting recovery. Please remember that not every therapy works for every child, and interviewing the different options available may be the only way to select an appropriate therapy for your child. You're best equipped to choose because you know your child best. Ask yourself: What can your child tolerate, and what is the benefit?

Chapter 12: FAQ

In caring for these children personally, I can tell you that a physician cannot see them for fifteen minutes and give quality care or gather any sufficient data. This work takes time, diligence, and patience from the doctor and the family. There is no miracle out there, but improvement and recovery are possible. As always, interview the person you are thinking of seeing to make sure they are the best fit for your child's medical team. It's not all about the formality; sometimes it's about faith in healing and knowing in your gut that you have found the most nurturing place for your child to heal.

To help guide you as you start your journey to optimal wellness, here are questions I am frequently asked:

Who can help me?

This becomes a philosophical decision for some. Ask yourself: What do I believe will help my child? What have other parents tried with success? Am I ready, able, and willing to commit to care? Every parent is committed to their child's health, but this is no walk in the park. The parents who have traveled down this road can tell you it is time-consuming and takes a commitment in every way. This is where the reality of what you can do meets your road of options.

Options include medications, therapy (applied behavior analysis, speech, occupational, CST, etc.), or a multi-disciplinary approach mixing the biomedical treatments and therapies together. I find it most advantageous to have a physician overseeing your child medically while getting the benefits of therapy too. If you find the right physician, then the team can work together for faster results. Whichever you choose, you must believe in the treatment approach you take and comply with whatever you opt to do to reap the maximum benefit.

Can I try more than one thing at a time?

Yes, if your doctor is taking care of the biomedical issues, then therapy can be that much more beneficial; the two can be synergistic. Most often, parents report that goals are being reached faster and improvements seem greater with a comprehensive treatment plan. Unfortunately, I have seen therapy providers that request a child drop all other treatments so they can gauge "what is working." While I see the logic in this isolation, sometimes this approach means years of trying one thing at a time, and time is too precious to risk. If your child recovers, do you really care what percentage was due to therapy vs. biomedical treatment? My advice for parents is to make sure each provider knows the treatment goals and that all are on the same page; this will keep you from wasting valuable time and finances.

How do I know if someone is qualified?

When faced with a developmentally delayed child, it is best for you to seek out a medical provider who specializes in children and has experience treating your child's specific delay. This may seem basic, but many providers see a variety of people from children to adults, which may equal less experience with your specific situation. Speaking to them or their nurse may help gauge if their expertise is a good fit for you. To put it simply, if you had a foot injury, you wouldn't call a gynecologist, right? Every day decisions have to be made, but they should not be made without all the facts, especially when it comes to medical care. Your child will have better results if you get the proper team in place.

What do I ask candidates for my child's treatment team?

First, you must write down the goals you have for your child and make sure the provider has direct experience achieving the results you are looking for. Of course no one can predict the future, but potential providers can tell you their experiences as they relate to similar situations and your child's condition, giving you a good idea of how they can or can't help. You must make the decision on who you feel can help you and your child reach your recovery goals.

Special needs children are the hardest hit by pathogenic yeast (Candida). Why?

These kids have weakened immune systems and abnormal detoxification systems that are fragile. Many have had tens of rounds of antibiotics to treat their recurring illness. There are many reasons a child may have pathogenic yeast, and the most common way a child gets it is by antibiotic use. The antibiotics go into the system and eliminate all the good bacteria with the bad, leaving an imbalance in the gut. Candida then multiply and populate the digestive tract, and this growth can take years to become symptomatic. In many cases when I trace through a child's infancy, symptom progression, and medication use, it's clear that the child has had an overgrowth of yeast for most of their lives.

How common is systemic Candida?

This is an epidemic I see in my practice, with over 75% of kids tested showing positive for pathogenic yeast.

What are the symptoms of Candida?

The symptoms range by age, exposure, and other underlying medical issues. Some symptoms may include bloating, gas, constipation, unresolved bed wetting, OCD, foul smelling stool, inappropriate laughing, eczema, bed-wetting, intermittent aggression, and poor behaviors that are unexplained. With aggression, most parents seek answers when they receive multiple complaints from school or have an inability to control their child at home. Just know that the symptoms don't have to be plentiful; your child can have just one.

How can parents determine if their child has a problem with yeast?

If your child is experiencing any of the symptoms above, then it's best to consult with someone immediately to see if testing is necessary. Your child can have only one of the symptoms and have yeast. The fact is that yeast doesn't go away on its own; it just grows and gets worse. Parents need to seek out care with a biomedical doctor or biomedical nutritionist. They will perform stool and urine testing to determine if yeast is present, and this will also reveal many other details necessary for treatment. Not every stool test is the same, so your pediatrician may not order the correct one. To detect yeast, you need a specialty test, and most biomedical doctors know how to perform these and interpret the results. Using an experienced biomedical doctor will ensure that you don't waste time or money.

If my child has yeast, how is it treated?

If yeast is present, I have found it best to attack it from a variety of ways, with treatment lasting for approximately four months. The test results will outline proper medications for the elimination of the specific species of yeast that tested positive. Variety in treatment helps to eliminate all the subtypes of yeast that are present. Also, be aware that not all prescription antifungals are the same, and in my experience very few pediatricians understand this difference. It's important to educate your child's pediatrician at every corner. Don't be afraid to tell them how great your kid is doing when you see the results—it brings power to the treatment and education to the forefront.

What can parents do to maintain healthy gut flora and yeast levels once they get their child's yeast under control?

There are many things that doctors need to clear up when yeast is discovered. Like I said before, it doesn't travel alone. The best way to keep it at bay long-term is to make sure the digestive system is healed, healthy, and kept in line with any dietary recommendations made by your doctor. Probiotics can also be helpful when using quality products. Lastly, find a way to keep your child healthy throughout the year to avoid the use of antibiotics that may spawn a new growth of yeast. If your child's medical team is focused on quality care and healing your child from the inside out, then much of this is not a concern.

What should parents expect after treatment?

I see and talk with parents all the time, whether in my office or when I am speaking publically, and they often say, "We are going to wait to see what happens for a while." This is playing with fire. Yeast doesn't go away. It grows and gets much worse, taking over the digestive system and causing immense inflammation that impairs your child neurologically. Many parents see a regression in symptoms within the first week of treatment, and in the long-term, they see additional strides made in therapy and at school.

Does the type of testing matter?

Remember that each doctor has a toolbox of testing that they use, and all are not equal. Neither is the interpretation of the results. Testing matters, and there are many wonderful companies out there that cater to special needs and developmentally delayed children. For example, many parents come to me with loads of prior testing, and I still find necessary testing missing or overlooked. In order to ensure proper testing is ordered, find someone who treats and sees children with special needs, and make sure they have the knowledge and experience in functional medicine and/or biomedical care (treating the core issues).

I have tried some biomedical recommendations I found online and saw no changes. What happened?

Well, no child is the same, and I think everyone can agree that's a fact. With biomedical interventions, treatment is truly personalized as each child is an individual and has unique challenges. Parents may decide to try to do things on their own without proper testing, and this is often a shot in the dark, limiting the child from reaching his or her full potential. Some families attempt dietary changes without seeking medical advice, and most are unable to stay consistent or are not following the diets correctly. The dietary changes can be made successfully with guidance, and when followed correctly, they can make a huge impact. Supplements are another big part of biomedical care, and parents might see, read, or hear about a product and decide to use it based on limited information. It is important to note that not all supplements or companies are the same. Many of these supplement companies are not overseen for their labeled efficacy, so the results may not be what you are hoping for. Many quality supplements can only be ordered by a physician; this makes a difference in effectiveness of the product and, in turn, your result. If you are going to spend the money on getting supplements for your child, then it's best to use products that you know will make a difference.

Is it safe for me to offer supplements to my child on my own?

In general, this issue is not about safety because most people give low doses of supplements that have low efficacy. However, it is possible to do more damage than good when you don't know what your child's underlying medical issues may be. The cost of supplements add up financially, and when you don't know exactly what to do, it gets expensive, frustrating, and can give you a false sense that biomedical interventions don't work. The largest risk is your child's possible recovery. It is best to get help from a physician; this will save money and time in the long run, not to mention will get your child on the road to healing.

Is there an age when treatment doesn't work any longer?

No, this is a common misunderstanding. Mixing supplements and making dietary changes is easier with a small child, but only because they don't fuss as much as a teen. As kids get older, there are just different obstacles to overcome. I always tell parents to get their child under care as soon as they can because I find the greatest, quickest results occur with younger children. I use the analogy that there is less garbage to clean up at three years old as compared to twelve years old—not to mention the difficulties getting compliance with the older kids. Nothing is impossible; it just takes knowing how to appeal to an older child to get them to want to help with their treatment and healing process.

How long does it take to get results?

The results vary by severity of symptoms, underlying medical issues, and compliance of care. I cannot stress enough to parents that consistency is the key to getting your child back on track. There are parents out there who jump from doctor to doctor and spend precious time they can never get back. Please don't make this mistake. You need to find a team, agree upon a treatment plan, and stick it out to get results. Some parents see dramatic results in weeks, and other families make small leaps over months. Either way, the common thread is consistency. This marathon is run together, and it has to be done safely and effectively to get the results you hope for your child.

Chapter 13: Common Poisons

There is no denying that environmental poisons exist. This becomes especially important when it affects a fragile developing child or a pregnant woman carrying her unborn child. I want to outline some facts as well as sources of aluminum, cadmium, arsenic, lead, mercury, and aspartame for you to be aware of. These are things you can begin avoiding immediately and, in turn, decrease your toxic load. It is important to note that within these lists will be common household items that you may need to research further on your own. For example, no two laundry detergents are the same, so use this as a guide to know when to look more closely at ingredient lists.

Toxic Elements

Aluminum, cadmium, arsenic, lead, and mercury are all elements that are found in everyday items and in the environment. I will outline some sources in tables for each of the elements, and you can use this as a quick reference to go around your home and make changes as needed.

Aluminum sources:

Vaccines	Aluminum cookware and utensils	Baking powder (Aluminum sulfate)
Antacids (some brands)	Antiperspirant	Aluminum cans
Drinking water	Dairy products	Pickled foods
Nasal spray	Toothpaste	Ceramics
Dental amalgams	Cigarette filters	Tobacco smoke
Rat poison	Pesticides	FD&C color additives
Vanilla powder	Table salt, some seasonings	Bleached flour
American cheese	Medicines with Kaolin	

Signs of Aluminum Toxicity: abnormal speech, involuntary jerks, osteomalacia (softening of bones), encephalopathy (disease of brain), Alzheimer's, and Parkinson's

Cadmium sources:

Drinking water	Refined wheat flour	Canned evaporated milk
Processed foods	Oysters	Organ meat (kidney & liver)
Cigarette smoke	Fertilizers	Paint pigments
Silver polish	Polyvinyl plastics	Rubber carpet backing
Nickel-cadmium batteries	Rust-proofing materials	

Signs of Cadmium Toxicity: upper leg pain, pain in low back, kidney problems, hypertension, vascular disease, and osteopenia (low bone density)

Arsenic sources:

Rat poison	Household detergent	Wood preservative
Insecticide residue on fruits and vegetables	Wine (if there's arsenic in pesticides used)	Colored chalk
Wallpaper dye and plaster	Drinking and sea water	Chicken (inorganic)
White rice (inorganic)		

Signs of Arsenic Toxicity: excessive protein in urine, hyperpigmentation, garlic breath odor, oral inflammation, and "rice-water" stool.

Lead sources:

Some red lipsticks	Some painted toys	Leaded house paint
Drinking water from lead pipes	Vegetables grown in contaminated lead soil	Boxed wine
Milk from animals grazing in lead fields	Bone meal	Certain Ayurvedic & Chinese herbs
Organ meat (liver)	Pesticides	Leaded caps on wine bottles
Painted pencils	Toothpaste	Newsprint
Colored printed materials	Eating utensils	Putty
Car batteries		

Signs of Lead Toxicity: anemia, kidney problems, anorexia, hypertension, muscle pain, constipation, metallic taste, and low IQ in children

Mercury sources:

Vaccines such as Thimerosal	Dental amalgams	Broken thermometers
Laxatives	Talc powder	Cosmetics
Latex paint	Fabric softeners	Suppositories
Floor wax and polish	Air conditioner filters	Wood preservatives
Certain batteries	Fungicides for lawn	Adhesives
Skin ointments		

Signs of Mercury Toxicity: insomnia, fatigue, poor short-term memory, tremor, oral inflammation, GI problems, kidney problems, and poor immune system

**Table information provided by Richard Lord (see appendix).

Aspartame

Aspartame is an artificial sweetener used in thousands of products, so it's easy to find in everyday foods. However, it is dangerous to consume as it contains chemicals that are toxic to our bodies. Many people have heard throughout the years about aspartame and its dangers; yet I find that many parents are still feeding it to their children unknowingly. It can be found everywhere, so let's get educated on what it is and how to avoid this common toxin going forward.

Combining two amino acids with methanol makes aspartame. The amino acids phenylalanine and aspartic acid are used, but when other amino acids aren't present, they become neurotoxic. More specifically, when aspartame is combined with the enzyme chymotrypsin in the small intestine, methanol is released and breaks down into formaldehyde (embalming fluid), a potent neurotoxin. Formaldehyde, methanol, phenylalanine, and aspartic acid all cause their own individual side effects. Formaldehyde is a known carcinogen that causes retinal damage, interferes with DNA replication, and causes birth defects. In the world of harmful food additives, aspartame may turn out to be the worst of them all. Collison et al. conducted a study where they reported that aspartame consumption impaired retention of learned behavior, contributed to blood glucose problems, and negatively impacted spatial learning and memory.

Building Blocks

Formaldehyde is found on the Environmental Protection Agency's list of hazardous chemicals and is also found in many vaccines, including the flu shot. The formaldehyde converts to formic acid, which is used as an activator to strip epoxy and urethane coatings.

Methanol is another component found in aspartame, and it is considered to be a cumulative poison. Methanol poisoning mostly causes vision problems, and due to the lack of certain enzymes, humans are more toxic to methanol than animals. The US Environmental Protection Agency considers a safe consumption of no more than 7.8mg per day. If you consume a one-liter beverage containing aspartame, your body creates seven times that amount. Each 12 oz. can of diet soda contains 200mg of aspartame and as much as 20mg of methanol. If you look closely, you will see a warning for phenylketanurics (PKU) on fake sugar packets. PKU is a rare condition; it's an inherited inability to break down phenylalanine, causing brain disorders, brain tumors, and birth defects. All babies are screened for PKU at birth.

Phenylalanine makes up 50% of aspartame and blocks the production of a neurotransmitter called serotonin, which may result in mood swings, depression, sleep disorders, intestinal problems, and poor appetite. Approximately 90% of the body's serotonin is located in the gut, so when aspartame is introduced, it interferes with the production of this very important neurotransmitter.

Aspartic acid makes up 40% of aspartame and can actually change DNA. In the 1970s scientists conducted aspartame research on lab animals and found that it caused holes in the brain, seizures, and death. There are several adverse reactions seen with aspartame ingestion, and many are still being discovered. The FDA reported that 75% of all complaints received about food additives are aspartame-related—that's 3 out of 4. The US Department of Health and Human Services released a list of 61 reported adverse reactions to aspartame, including:

- Chest pains
- Asthma
- Arthritis
- Migraine headaches
- Insomnia
- Seizures
- Tremors
- Vertigo
- Weight gain

Since aspartame is used in diet drinks and sugar-free foods, it's surprising to see weight gain on the list. According to a study by Yang, aspartame actually stimulates appetite and causes cravings for carbohydrates, causing weight gain over time.

Aspartame may be the unidentified environmental trigger for:

- Brain tumors
- Autoimmune diseases
- Migraine
- Mild to severe depression
- Abdominal pain
- Memory loss
- Epilepsy
- Insomnia
- Rash
- Anxiety/phobia disorders
- Tinnitus
- Fibromyalgia
- Numbness & tingling of extremities
- Confusion
- Attention deficit disorder (ADD and ADHD)

How do I get Aspartame out of my body?

It typically takes at least 60 days without any aspartame (NutraSweet) to see a significant improvement. Check **all** labels very carefully, including vitamins and pharmaceuticals. Look for the word "aspartame" or any of its pseudonyms (see below) on the label to avoid it.

What contains aspartame?

Aspartame is an artificial sweetener found in over 6,000 products including diet drinks, toothpaste, sugar-free products, sugar-free chewing gums, dietary supplements, sport drinks, energy drinks, and medications. Sugar-free = bad for you.

This is a list of alternate names for aspartame. Pay close attention as any of these names relate to all the above-mentioned data. No one ingredient listed below is better or worse than the other; they are all equally bad. Please avoid them all!

- Aspartame
- Acesulfame-k
- Sunette
- Acesulfame potassium
- Phenylketanurics
- N-L-alpha-Aspartyl-L-phenylalanine 1-methyl ester
- 3-Amino-N-(alpha-carboxyphenethyl) Succinamic acid N-methyl ester
- APM
- SC-18862
- Canderel™
- Equal™
- Diketopiperazine, or DKP (This known brain tumor agent is a breakdown product of aspartame.)
- NutraSweet™ (not always listed clearly on the ingredient label)

Pregnancy & Aspartame

I am sure after reading about aspartame that many of you, especially those who are pregnant, will refrain. That said, I want to explain why this chemical is especially dangerous for pregnancy. A woman's metabolism is dramatically altered by pregnancy. Many women are weight-conscious during their pregnancy and are likely to consume large amounts of these low-calorie products in an effort to limit weight gain. However, product labeling does not include the amount of aspartame in the product or any warning other than for phenylketonurics (PKU). One in every fifty people carries the gene for PKU even though they do not have the disorder themselves. PKU is an inherited disorder that does not allow the body to metabolize phenylalanine (a component of aspartame). This causes excess build-up in the bloodstream, which can cause retardation. If a woman who carries the PKU gene procreates with a man who also carries that recessive gene, she could give birth to a baby with the condition. If she then consumes too much aspartame during pregnancy, her baby could be born with developmental issues, specifically neurological conditions.

When a woman ingests too much aspartame during pregnancy, her blood plasma concentrations of phenylalanine can rise up to 2.5 times, creating an imbalance. The placenta will magnify this imbalance another two-fold, and the baby's blood brain barrier (BBB) will magnify it yet another two times. This is a total of 6 times the phenylalanine concentration, significantly raising the risk of mental retardation. Many mothers ask, "How much is too much?" Studies show that 34mg, or seven diet sodas, doubles the plasma phenylalanine concentrations.

Newborns & Aspartame

The aspartic acid in aspartame is a neurotoxin in high concentrations and poses a significant hazard to the developing nervous system, penetrating the BBB, causing brain tumors, abscesses, and death of brain cells.

Children/Teens & Aspartame

Those children exposed to aspartame during fetal development may have alterations in brain development that could later result in such serious brain disorders as autism, learning differences, hyperactivity, and schizophrenia. By age four, the brain has reached 80% of its adult weight, and by age sixteen, the brain is full-size although not fully developed. The brain development and new connections continue to mature for long periods of time, making teenagers potentially vulnerable to the effects of aspartame. The onset of these behavioral and learning disorders may not show up immediately, but rather may be delayed for many years following birth because of the timing of the onset of specialized brain functions. For example, damaged speech areas of the brain would not be evident in a newborn baby, but would be evident when the child began to learn to speak.

As children age and become teens, they begin to make food decisions away from home while out with friends and at school. Most chewing gum, sodas, sports drinks, and snack items contain aspartame. I often find that teens who have trouble with attention, focus, or behavior are getting loads of aspartame in their diets, so it is best to educate your teen about not only what to avoid but *why* they need to avoid it. Most teens will listen when you explain the reason behind what you are requesting. If it seems to them like you are dictating unreasonable commands, they won't listen. But if you recruit them to work together to better their health, teens will usually do what's best.

The common poisons discussed in this section are things most people can refrain from. This information can empower parents to help their children at home, regardless of age or gender. Nobody will refute the scientific data, but many still argue, "Does this really contribute to abnormal development?" Well, what do you think—should you take the chance? Why use products that could potentially damage development when alternatives exist? A little awareness is usually all that's needed; simple education can help parents and children alike get on the right track and stay there.

Chapter 14:
Treating at Home – Common Remedies

Most of us were brought up with our mothers and grandmothers using their own remedies at home to make us feel better, and regardless of the many advances in medicine, this continues to be something mothers should do for their children. The following are some common things you can do at home to help your child fight and even prevent illness.

This information is not intended to provide medical advice, diagnosis, or treatment. Content is for informational purposes only and is not intended to be a substitute for professional medical care. Please seek the advice of your physician or other qualified health provider with any questions you may have regarding your child's medical condition.

Colic
Colic typically manifests within the first few weeks, and as discussed in this book, the best way to eliminate this is craniosacral therapy (CST). While you wait to find a provider to help you and your infant, you can try a few things that may help you manage at home:

Nutritional Supplements:

- Use Hyland's colic tablets or gripe water as directed. This helps about 50% of children and is worth a try.
- Improper digestion can be a contributing factor. Mom needs to take digestive enzymes as directed to help aid digestion. Many mothers only figure out their digestion issues and/or food allergies once they have a baby. Infants have a much more sensitive system and are a good gauge.
- For constipation, stay hydrated and introduce a probiotic for both mother and baby. Make sure to use an infant probiotic for your child.

Dietary Recommendations:

- Remove dairy from the mother's diet or switch from dairy-based formula.
- Gas and constipation are common issues with a colicky baby. Reduce gas-producing foods via mother's diet, consuming at least 80% cooked food and only 20% uncooked or raw foods.
- Remove caffeine from mother's diet (yes, this includes chocolate).

General Recommendations:

- Call your lactation consultant to make sure there are no unresolved issues with feeding that are causing the baby frustration or hunger.
- Try sleeping the infant on an angle in case they are having a small amount of reflux, a symptom that will also be alleviated with CST.
- Try a warm Epsom salt bath to help relax them.
- Relax—with the new baby coming home, the atmosphere can be very tense. Children pick up on all that energy and stress, which causes worsening of the problem.

Prevention:

- A chiropractic wellness visit shortly after birth will alleviate the potential problems that may lead to colic. I tend to see colic begin between four and six weeks, so get an appointment as soon as you are ready to leave the house after birth.

Common Cold

Most every child gets a cold at some point, especially daycare and school-aged kids. This is a virus that affects the respiratory tract and gives symptoms of stuffy nose, cough, ear pain, sore throat, and sinus discomfort, to name the most common. There is no cure for a cold, so the goal is to minimize the symptoms and discomfort until the child's body gets over it. Taking an antibiotic is often ineffective unless there is a bacterial infection (ear or sinus); even then, with early intervention an antibiotic can be avoided.

Nutritional Supplements:

- Briar Rose is used for acute illness, given 2–3 times per day while acute and twice weekly for an immune boost through winter.
- Colloidal silver liquid is a natural antibiotic and can be used if you suspect a bacterial infection. Use several sprays by mouth 2–3 times per day. There is no need to mix this with anything; deliver straight and have your infant swallow.
- Coldcalm by Boiron can help with sneezing, runny nose, nasal congestion, and minor sore throat. This should be used for children over 3 years as directed and can be purchased at most health food stores.
- Hyland's cold tablets are homeopathic tablets designed to help with common cold symptoms. These can be used for children over 6 months of age as directed and can be purchased at most grocery

stores, Wal-Mart, and Target.
- Immune boosters (see *Immune Boost* below)
    - Nutraceutical supplements can be ordered by your doctor. These are natural medicines made in a medical-grade facility, overseen for quality and content of ingredients. There is no body governing many of the supplements carried at the store, but a doctor can order these higher quality supplements. If you are going to spend the money on supplementation, you should get something that will work and is of high quality.

Dietary Recommendations:
- Increase water intake, giving as much as your child will drink throughout the entire day.
- Clear soups are easier for the body during this time as they do not contribute to excessive secretions.
- Remove all sugars as they suppress the immune system and may slow the immune response.
- Avoid dairy, which is mucus-producing.

General Recommendations:
- See your chiropractor immediately for symptom relief. Nothing will help more, and they can suggest additional treatment options.
- Increase fluids and rest.
- Congestion can be really difficult and can interfere with sleep and appetite.
    o For infants, suction out the mucus from their nose to alleviate build up and congestion.
    o Saline spray can help break up the crusty nose of any child.
    o In older children, sinus flushing with saline can help break

up the mucus. Have them blow their nose after each flush.

o A humidifier is always good to have around the house. You can try leaving it on overnight to see if that helps break up congestion.

o All ages can benefit from a steamy bathroom. It helps with congestion and chest coughs. I instruct parents to turn on a super-hot shower, close the bathroom door, and let the room get steamy. When it's ready, take the child in there to play or feed.

Prevention:

- Regular chiropractic care keeps alignment optimal and decreases chances of illness.
- Muco-coccinum is a homeopathic cold prevention option for children 2 and up. You will place 1 tablet under the tongue and let it dissolve (does not taste bad) every 2 weeks through the cold and flu season. For cold or flu treatment, increase to daily doses, not exceeding 3 doses in 24 hours.
- Stick to an immune protocol during the start of school and during cold and flu season.

Constipation

I have already discussed constipation in detail, so make sure you review the information in Chapter 7: Four Red Flags. The goal is to have normal bowel movements daily, so take a look at the list below to see what you can do to make adjustments. If these do not work, please seek help from a biomedical or functional medicine doctor to rule out leaky gut, yeast overgrowth, or impaction. Keep in mind that, although rare, the first symptom of botulism in infants is usually constipation. If your infant has severe or difficult to treat constipation, especially if he or she also has other symptoms like weakness and poor muscle tone, ask your doctor about botulism.

Nutritional Supplements:

- Remove foods discussed in Chapter 2: Early Interventions in Infancy.

- Dehydration can lead to constipation. Increase fluids during this time.

- Increase fiber via supplementation or food. If a child is eating solids and has constipation, try strained prunes, apricots, or spinach. For infants who are not yet eating solids, the mother can take fiber.

- Food grade aloe vera juice or capsules are fast-acting and usually mild in taste when mixed with coconut kefir or a small portion of applesauce. You can dose 1 teaspoon 1–3 times daily. I recommend starting with 1 teaspoon and seeing what happens, then increasing as needed. Please note that not all aloe supplements are the same in potency and preparation, so get a recommendation if you have questions about efficacy. This can be a potent laxative, causing cramping and diarrhea, so I recommend using it for children above age 3. The maximum dose is that which produces stools that are too loose.

- Vitamin C can be given in doses of 500–3000mg 1–3 times daily. The buffered form is the best and can be very effective in moving bowels. You can start with a small dose and increase as needed. The maximum dose is that which produces stools that are too loose.

- Magnesium citrate is the most effective and gentle way to move the bowels. The daily dose is 4mg per pound. For example, a 30-pound child should take 120mg of magnesium daily, so if your child is constipated, you can give more. You will want to give 2/3 of the daily dose at bedtime and the remaining 1/3 in the morning. If your child is not on magnesium daily, then start with the daily dose. The upper limit not to be exceeded is 350mg. The maximum dose for any child is that which produces stools that are too loose.

- Probiotics are great for daily intake and can help in these times too. Give as directed. Make sure to buy a refrigerated option with the highest amount of cultures per capsule and that has the greatest variety of cultures.

Dietary Recommendations:
- Increase fiber via supplementation or food. If a child is eating solids and has constipation, try strained prunes, apricots, or spinach. For infants who are not yet eating solids, the mother can take fiber.
- Decrease foods that tend to be more binding, such as cow milk, soy, cheese, yogurt, cooked carrots, and bananas.

General Recommendations:
- A chiropractic adjustment can provide relief. When the pelvis or sacrum is subluxated, the nerves that go to the digestive system are affected, and constipation can be the result.
- Abdominal massage can be helpful. Make sure to use a lubricant such as lotion for comfort. Massage the entire abdomen (in a clockwise direction) gently starting at the right lower abdomen up to the rib cage and across to the left and back down the left side. Then begin this sequence again, following the intestine in one large circular pattern, ONLY in a clockwise direction.
- Epsom salt baths are relaxing and increase circulation of the intestines. Epsom salt is magnesium sulfate, and most times after a bath, children will have a bowel movement.
- Enemas, suppositories, and medicinal laxatives do <u>not</u> go on this list for me. If it comes to this, you very much need guidance and should seek help instead of performing these treatments at home. I know many people recommend them, but these are short-term fixes and often leave parents ignoring the bigger issues.

Prevention:

- Regular chiropractic care will keep the body in balance and free of subluxations. When the pelvis or sacrum is subluxated, the nerves that go to the digestive system are affected, and constipation can be the result. A simple visit to the chiropractor can keep your child regular.
- Maintain a healthy diet that's free of cow dairy and soy products and that's balanced with vegetables and good gluten-free fiber sources.
- Daily administration of a probiotic is highly recommended. The type of probiotic should be switched every 3–4 months to make sure varied cultures are getting into the body. Not every probiotic is made the same.

Ear Infection

This is one of the most common things parents will face, but when caught early, is one of the most treatable at home. Infants tend to be at higher risk for ear infections due to simple anatomy. The eustachian tube in an infant is horizontal, unlike an older child or adult whose eustachian tube is vertical. The horizontal positioning makes it harder for drainage and easier for bacteria to get caught and cause an infection. My recommendation is to always call your chiropractor first because they can help with drainage, which is the reason why there is an infection. They'll also examine the ear for progress or regression, help walk you through natural options, and make sure the infection doesn't keep recurring.

Nutritional Supplements:

- Natural ear drops can be found at most health food stores, and there are many manufacturers on the market. The natural ear drops will contain many ingredients, but the most important is garlic. You want to look for the manufacturer brand that has the highest garlic content; these are typically oil-based and really soothe the pain and discomfort associated with an ear infection. Garlic is a natural antibiotic. You will want to administer to both ears, using these drops several times a day and making sure the liquid stays inside the ear (not on a cotton swab). Have your child lie down on their side, drop 3–5 drops into the ear, let the solution sit inside for 15 minutes if possible, and then switch sides and repeat. You may want to run the dropper under warm water to help warm the liquid; this can help if fever is associated as the inside of the ear is very hot and the drops may be cold. Also note that these drops are odorous and do stain fabric, so you may want to protect the pillow your child is lying on with a towel to avoid staining.

- Lavender and tea tree oil can be used as a foot rub. Combine one part lavender and one part melaleuca (tea tree) oil and dilute with olive oil or another household base oil. Once combined, lather the feet in the oil; covering feet with socks is optional.

- Vitamin C can be given in doses of 500–3000mg 1–3 times daily. The buffered form is the best. You can start with a small dose and increase as needed. The maximum dose is that which produces stools that are too loose.

- Colloidal silver liquid is a natural antibiotic and can be used if you suspect a bacterial infection. Use several sprays by mouth 2–3 times per day. There is no need to mix this with anything; deliver straight and have your child swallow. You can also use 2–3 drops directly in the ears, using the same guidelines as the natural ear drops above.

- Probiotics can initially be taken daily, and when healthy, doses can be weaned down to 3–4 times weekly. I suggest switching probiotic brands at least three times per year to make sure enough variety in cultures is achieved.

Dietary Recommendations:

- Increase water intake, giving as much as your child will drink throughout the entire day.
- Clear soups are easier for the body during this time as they do not contribute to excessive secretions.
- Remove all sugars as they suppress the immune system and may slow the immune response.
- Avoid dairy, which is mucus-producing.

General Recommendations:

- See your chiropractor immediately for symptom relief. Nothing will help more, and they can suggest additional treatment options.
- Craniosacral therapy (CST) can alleviate restrictions and improve drainage, minimizing the chances of chronic infections.
- Try to keep your infant elevated while feeding and during the day to keep fluid from collecting in the ears.

Prevention:

- Regular chiropractic care keeps alignment optimal and decreases chances of illness.
- Regular CST sessions can keep restrictions from occurring and decrease the occurrence of infections.

Fever

A fever can be good news for your child because this means their body is fighting an illness. A bacteria or virus does not survive well under increased temperatures, so the body naturally increases its temperature to kill off these offenders. A child's temperature can be affected by physical activity, stress, clothing, weather, and time of day, so make sure to keep an eye on temperature and retake it if you think one of these variables is a factor. Closely monitor your child, as always, and pay special attention to appetite, fluid intake, exposure to bites, infection, food, or environmental allergy. Observe your child during this time and ask the following: How ill do they seem? Are there any other signs like poor appetite, irritability, rash, or another unusual component? If you notice anything out of the ordinary, medical care may be necessary to rule out a more serious cause. A slight fever can be dealt with at home, and no intervention is necessary to reduce it. If the fever gets above 102 degrees Fahrenheit, a fever-reducing medication may be in order. I like to have parents try to treat as much at home and let a fever break on its own; this of course will be for you decide based on the above variables.

Nutritional Supplements:
- Vitamin C can be given in doses of 500-3000mg 1–3 times daily. The buffered form is the best. You can start with a small dose and increase as needed. The maximum dose is that which produces stools that are too loose.
- Rub peppermint oil on the feet, diluted with olive oil or another household base oil.
- Immune system booster (see *Immune boost* below)

Dietary Recommendations:
- Increase water intake, giving as much as your child will drink throughout the entire day.

General Recommendations:
- Draw a tepid bath using 1–2 cups of Epsom salt, depending on how full the tub is.
- Wrap the calves in socks or a cloth soaked in lemon juice, which can

bring down a fever. To prepare, heat a cup of water with the juice of one lemon until it is almost boiling. Soak the cloth or sock and allow it to cool to a warm temperature before placing it on your child's calves. Wrap each calf, cover with dry socks or cloth to lock in the warmth, and cover the calves with a blanket for 20 minutes. You can do this 1–3 times daily.

- Keep your child in comfortable light clothing and under a light sheet. Make sure to have a blanket close in case they get cold or begin to shiver.
- Visit your chiropractor. Many times a chiropractic adjustment will drop a fever that same day.

Homeopathic Options:

Homeopathy can be very helpful, but does follow rules, so read through the symptoms associated with the fever to decide on the best treatment for your child. These can be very effective and should reduce a fever within hours. The following remedies can be bought at your local market (e.g., Whole Foods) or nutrition store. <u>Do not give more than one remedy at a time</u>. If your child is not responding, you can discontinue it and try another remedy. Please do not administer any of the homeopathic remedies with other medications, even with over-the-counter (OTC) fever reducers. If two remedies fail, call your child's doctor.

Aconite:

Used for the very beginning stages of a fever, which may come on after being out in cold weather. The child may be apprehensive and anxious, but should not be experiencing fever sweats.

Dose: 12c or 30c, given every 2–3 hours until the fever breaks. Children are generally better by the third dose. If no improvement after that, switch remedies.

Arsenicum album:

Used for a fever that increases between midnight and 2 a.m. and for children who are anxious, fidgety, and reporting leg pain. A cold compress and blankets on the legs may help.

Dose: 9c or 30x, given once every 2 hours for a total of 4 doses maximum

Belladonna:

Used for sudden high fever presenting with sweating, chills, flushed face, and dilated pupils. The child may be fearful and find noise and sound bothersome.

Dose: 12c or 30c given every 2–3 hours for 4 doses or until fever breaks, whichever comes first. Children are generally better by the third dose.

Drug interactions with acetaminophen (Tylenol), chlorpheniramine, pseudoephedrine, Zyrtec, Alka-Seltzer Cold and Cough, Pediacof, Robitussin, Benadryl, and other allergy and cold meds. To be safe, do not administer belladonna with any other medications without consulting a doctor.

Bryonia:

Used for fever seen with irritability, strong thirst, and possible constipation. The child generally wants to be left alone.

Dose: 30x or 9c, given once every 2 hours for a total of 4 doses maximum

Chamomilla:

Used for fever associated with teething, or when the child feels worse with heat, under a blanket, and at night.

Dose: 12x or 6c, given every 2 hours for up to 3 doses. Once the cheeks are no longer red, you can return to using ferrum phoshoricum every 2 hours up to 6 doses. See below for potencies.

Ferrum Phosphoricum:
Used for moderate fever onset and fevers of low degree. Child is not appearing sick.
Dose: 9c or 12x, given every 2–3 hours for a total of 6 doses or until fever breaks, whichever comes first. Children are generally better by the third dose.

Prevention:
Regular chiropractic care keeps alignment optimal and decreases chances of illness.

Flu

The flu is a virus that structurally changes, and therefore it's hard to immunize against it. It is common to alleviate the symptoms of the flu, which may include fever, achiness, chills, fatigue, and lessening of appetite. The flu passes within days but can be miserable, so the following things may help to increase comfort.

Nutritional Supplements:
- Reduce fever if needed. (see *Fever*)
- Vitamin C can be given in doses of 500–3000mg 1–3 times daily. The buffered form is the best. You can start with a small dose and increase as needed. The maximum dose is that which produces stools that are too loose.

- Nutraceutical supplements can be ordered by your doctor. These are natural medicines made in a medical-grade facility, overseen for quality and content of ingredients. There is no body governing many of the supplements carried at the store, but a doctor can order these higher quality supplements. If you are going to spend the money on supplementation, you should get something that will work and is of high quality.

Dietary Recommendations:
- Increase water intake, giving as much as your child will drink throughout the entire day.
- Clear soups are easier for the body during this time as they do not contribute to excessive secretions.
- Remove all sugars as they suppress the immune system and may slow the immune response.
- Avoid dairy, which is mucus-producing.

General Recommendations:
- See your chiropractor immediately for symptom relief. Nothing will help more, and they can suggest additional treatment options.
- Increase fluids and rest.

Prevention:
- Regular chiropractic care keeps alignment optimal and decreases chances of illness.
- Muco-coccinum by Unda can be found at most health food stores. For ages 2 and up, give 1 tablet every 2 weeks during flu season.
- See *Immune* recommendations, and keep your kids on supplements throughout flu season.

Headache

Children hardly ever have headaches, so any headache should be taken seriously. They can get them from physical activity, injury, food allergy, and just being a rough and tumble kid, but periodically these can also be bigger medical concerns. It is difficult for kids to explain their symptoms, so try some of the following treatments. It never hurts to call and make an appointment with your chiropractor; many times a simple adjustment can alleviate the headache the same day.

Nutritional Supplements:
- Calcium/Magnesium citrate calms the system down and relaxes the blood vessels. You should be able to find liquid and capsule options. Use as directed by your doctor.
- Omega fatty acids should be a daily routine for children. Consult with your doctor about options as there are many poor quality brands on the market.

Dietary Recommendations:
- This might seem too easy, but just make sure your child has eaten. Sometimes kids get so busy that they forget to eat, causing their blood sugar to plummet, giving them a headache.
- Drink water. Dehydration headaches occur pretty frequently due to inadequate intake of fluids.
- The headache diet is geared to eliminate irritants in food. Avoid fat, dairy, beans, olives, pickles, chocolate, sweets, artificial sweeteners, processed meats such as hot dogs and sausage, caffeine, MSG (look at labels), and any known food allergies until headaches subside. If headaches are more frequent, then consider food allergy testing with your child's doctor.

General Recommendations:

- See your chiropractor immediately. Nothing will help more, and they can suggest additional treatment options
- Natural oils, such as peppermint, can be used to rub on the temples.
- Help your child relax. It's amazing how much stress they put on children in school these days, and this may lead to tension. Offer your best tender loving care to help your child through it.
- Epsom salt baths are relaxing and will help soothe tension in their muscles.

Prevention:

- Regular chiropractic care keeps alignment optimal and decreases chances of muscle tension, headaches, and pain.
- Make sure your children are eating enough protein and have snacks on hand so they can keep their blood sugar up.
- Remove caffeine, sugars, and nightshade foods (e.g., potatoes, bell peppers, eggplant).
- Ensure your child gets plenty of sleep.

Immune Boost

Pick one or two from this list to give depending on age and tolerance of your child. These immune boosters can be used when illness comes on and also as a preventative measure when your child has been exposed to someone who's sick.

- Vitamin C can be given in doses of 500–3000mg 1–3 times daily. The buffered form is the best. You can start with a small dose and increase as needed. The maximum dose is that which produces stools that are too loose.
- A vitamin/mineral blend will contain all the essentials the body

needs for healing. These should be given daily anyway.

- Grapefruit seed extract is a great natural antibiotic and antifungal. This liquid magic is not tasty, but when mixed with a very small portion of orange juice can be drawn into a syringe and easily given. Dose 1–5 drops 2–3 times daily while sick.

- Garlic given as a supplement can be a very powerful natural antibiotic and anti-inflammatory. The dose is 1–2 pills or the liquid equivalent.

- MCT liquid is a natural antibiotic and antifungal and has a very mild taste, which makes it easy to administer to any child. The dose is 1 tablespoon 2 times daily.

- Briar Rose is used for acute illness, infections, ear infections, and sore throats, among other ailments. Give 2–3 times per day while acute and twice weekly for immune boosts through winter.

- Probiotics can initially be taken daily and, when healthy, can be weaned down to 3–4 times weekly. I suggest switching probiotic brands at least three times per year to make sure enough variety in cultures is achieved.

- Omega fatty acids should be a daily routine for children. Consult with your doctor about options as there are many poor quality brands on the market.

- Nutraceutical supplements can be ordered by your doctor. These are natural medicines made in a medical-grade facility, overseen for quality and content of ingredients. There is no body governing many of the supplements carried at the store, but a doctor can order these higher quality supplements. If you are going to spend the money on supplementation, you should get something that will work and is of high quality.

Sore Throat

A sore throat can be miserable, making it hard to sleep and eat. Start treating at home at the first signs of a sore throat. Keep a close eye on your child as this may be a strep infection, which your doctor can help you treat naturally. The pediatrician will perform a throat culture to identify streptococcus, BUT this test may come back negative even when children have strep. So, if treatment doesn't resolve the problem or you swear based on experience that your child has strep, then insist on a blood test. If an antibiotic is suggested, wait three days to allow the acute portion of the strep to pass. Research suggests that the chances of reinfection lessen if you wait three days, allowing the body to defend itself the way it is designed to do (see *Journal of Pediatric Infectious Disease* for more information). In the meantime, use some of the natural approaches listed to get them through that three days and see what the blood results yield; if strep is negative on a blood test, then there's no need to use an antibiotic because the cause is viral and an antibiotic will be ineffective. You may also want to discuss an antibiotic injection option for treatment, which does not require ingestion of an antibiotic. I have gone through what oral antibiotics do to the body in this book, so think carefully before choosing this option. If strep is recurring, request blood tests to confirm; your child's health is on the line, so do not be afraid to insist. Recurring strep can lead to more serious complications such as PANDAS (pediatric autoimmune neuropsychiatric disorders associated with streptococcal infections) and in some cases needs aggressive treatment to rid the system of the entire infection. Not to mention ongoing strep infections can cause developmental delays, OCD behaviors, and tics.

Nutritional Supplements:
- Briar Rose is used for sore throats among other ailments. Give 2–3 times per day while acute and twice weekly for an immune boost through winter.
- Colloidal silver liquid is a natural antibiotic and can be used for a sore throat in spray or dropper form. You can use several sprays by mouth 2–3 times per day. It instantly soothes the throat, alleviating pain. The taste is very mild, so there is no need to mix it with anything; deliver straight, and have your child swallow to coat the entire throat.
- Immune boosters (see list) can be used to gargle for a sore throat, but it is also good to ingest them to boost the immune system.

Dietary Recommendations:
- Drink plenty of fluids.
- Make homemade popsicles from organic fruit juice in ice trays. Make sure you water down the juice because children do not need excess sugar while sick; it suppresses their immune system.
- Reduce sugars, dairy, and refined carbohydrates in foods and beverages while your child is ill. Their immune system will thank you for it.
- Warm non-caffeinated tea with lemon and honey can soothe a sore throat. This can be made to gargle or drink. You can add tincture (liquid) immune boosters to this too. Note: Honey should not be given to children under the age of one.

General Recommendations:
- A chiropractic adjustment is useful for lymphatic drainage and can alleviate additional illness from occurring, such as an ear or sinus infection and fever.
- Rest and keep your child away from other children and siblings.

Prevention:

- Regular chiropractic care will keep your child's body in balance and free of subluxations, giving it the ability to fight infection and remain healthy all year long.

Thrush

Thrush is a fungal infection (candidiasis) in the mouth and is very common for infants under six months of age. It appears as a white, flaky, almost curd-like patch covering some or the entire tongue, gums, interior cheeks, and lips. It is best not to pick off the patches or scrape them as this may cause further irritation and bleeding. Thrush can interfere with feeding and can cause nipples to be infected. It is best to contact your doctor if feeding decreases for more than a few days, your infant loses weight, or other symptoms develop such as fever, rash, reflux, or illness. It is important to treat this and make sure it is eliminated because it could lead to failure to thrive, chronic fungal infection, and dehydration.

Nutritional Supplements:

- Gentian violet can help clear thrush and can be swabbed inside the entire mouth and on mother's nipples. Treatment of the nipples is to make sure you don't keep giving it back and forth. This is violet in color and will stain everything it touches, so be aware.
- Caprylic acid (also called MCT), commonly found in foods such as coconut oil, is a potent natural anti-fungal. Studies have shown that dietary caprylic acid helps inhibit the growth of *Candida albicans* and other opportunistic fungi in both the small and large intestine. You can get this in pill form for a breastfeeding mother and in liquid form to give directly to an infant. The liquid has a very mild taste. Mothers should take caps as directed 2–3 times per day. For children,

the dose is 1/2–1 tablespoon 2 times daily depending on age (for infants, start with the smaller dose of 1/2 tablespoon).

- Probiotics can initially be taken daily, and when healthy, can be weaned down to 3–4 times weekly. I suggest switching probiotic brands at least three times per year to make sure enough variety in cultures is achieved. Make sure to use an infant probiotic formula when giving directly to your infant (under 12 months).

- Grapefruit seed extract (GSE) is a great natural antifungal and can be used on the surface as well as ingested to help with yeast. Make a mixture of 10 drops GSE to 1 ounce of distilled water, and administer by coating all affected areas of the mouth up to 6 times throughout the day. The use of distilled water to make your solution is very important because the chemicals placed in your local tap water to kill bacteria can reduce the effectiveness of the active ingredients in GSE. If thrush is not markedly improved by the second day, increase the mixture to 15 drops of GSE per 1 ounce of distilled water, and administer hourly throughout the day. If this does not seem to resolve the thrush, try another method or call your doctor.

  o Breastfeeding mothers will also need to use this solution with an absorbent swab on the nipples along with baby's mouth once every hour during all waking hours. Swab baby's mouth **prior** to nursing and mom's nipples **after** nursing. Applying it to baby's mouth prior to nursing will help them to avoid the possibility of baby associating the bitter taste with nursing.

  o If the diaper area is affected, put the same strength solution into a spray bottle or swab as above at every diaper change. If the area on their bottom is irritated and raw, you will want to skip this step as it may irritate or burn. Instead, keep the area moistened with calendula or another natural cream.

Dietary Recommendations:
- A breastfeeding mother needs to keep a low-sugar and low-carbohydrate diet because yeast (Candida) feeds on sugar.

General Recommendations:
- Avoid scraping the thrush off as this may irritate further or cause bleeding.

Prevention:
- Both mother and child should avoid taking antibiotics as this is the most common cause.
- Take a daily probiotic to maintain healthy gut flora and balance. Mother and baby both need to be taking this. For infants (under 12 months), make sure you are giving an infant probiotic formula.

References

About SPD resource page. Sensory Processing Foundation Web site. http://www. sinetwork.org/about-sensory-processing-disorder.html. Accessed May 2012.

Asperger Syndrome resources page. Kids Health Web site. http://kidshealth.org/ parent/medical/brain/asperger.html#. Accessed January 2012.

Atladóttir HO, Pedersen MG, Thorsen P, et al. Association of family history of autoimmune diseases and autism spectrum disorders. *Pediatrics.* 2009;2:687-94.

Collison KS, et al. Gender dimorphism in aspartame-induced impairment of spatial cognition and insulin sensitivity. *PLoS One.* 2012;7(4):e31570.

Could Your Baby Be Suffering from Food Allergy or Intolerance? ICPA Web site. http://icpa4kids.org/Wellness-Articles/could-your-baby-be-suffering-from-food-allergy-or-intolerance.html Published June 1, 2008. Accessed September 14, 2012.

Hassal E. Over-Prescription of Acid-Suppressing Medications in Infants: How It Came About, Why It's Wrong, and What to Do About It. *Journal of Pediatrics.* 2011;2:193-198.

Keil A, Daniels JL, Forssen U, et al. Parental autoimmune diseases associated with autism spectrum disorders in offspring. *Epidemiology.* 2010;6:805-808.

Leaky Gut resources. Leaky Gut Syndrome Web site. http://www.leakygut.co.uk. Accessed June 11, 2011.

Lord R, Bralley JA. *Laboratory Evaluations for Integrative and Functional Medicine.* 2nd edition. Duluth, GA: Metamatrix Institute; 2008.

McDermott M, McVicar K, Cohen H, et al. Gastrointestinal Symptoms in Children with an Autism Spectrum Disorder and Language Regression. *Pediatric Neurology.* 2008;39:392-398.

Mouridsen SE, Rich B, Isager T, et al. Autoimmune diseases in parents of children with infantile autism: a case-control study. *Dev Med Child Neurology.* 2007;6:429-32.

Ohm J. Breast to Bowl: Introducing Baby's First Foods. ICPA Web site. http://icpa4kids.org/Wellness-Articles/breast-to-bowl-introducing-babys-first-foods.html. Published October 7, 2008. Accessed September 14, 2012.

Oliver K. Rice Cereal vs. Real Food. Your Green Baby Web site. http://yourgreenbaby.ca/?p=380. Published October 18, 2010. Accessed September 2011.

Palmer L. When the Pediatrician Says GER. *Pathways Magazine.* 2008;18:12-16.

Wong K. Leaky Gut Syndrome/Intestinal Permeability resource page. Alternative Medicine Guide Web site. http://altmedicine.about.com/od/healthconditionsdisease/a/TestLeakyGut.htm. Updated July 23, 2007. Accessed June 11, 2011.

Yang Q. Gain weight by "going diet?" Artificial sweeteners and the neurobiology of sugar cravings. *Neuroscience.* 2010;83:101-108.

CPSIA information can be obtained at www.ICGtesting.com
Printed in the USA
LVOW100917031212

309781LV00003B/5/P